The

IVF

Blueprint

The

IVF

Blueprint

Everything You Need to Know
About **In Vitro Fertilization,**
Egg Freezing, and **Embryo Transfer**

· ·

Abby Eblen, MD, MSHS; Carrie Bedient, MD;
and Susan Hudson, MD, MBA

Little, Brown Spark
New York Boston London

Little, Brown Spark Hachette Book Group
1290 Avenue of the Americas, New York, NY 10104
littlebrownspark.com

First Edition: September 2025

Little, Brown Spark is an imprint of Little, Brown and Company, a division of Hachette Book Group, Inc. The Little, Brown Spark name and logo are trademarks of Hachette Book Group, Inc.

The publisher is not responsible for websites (or their content) that are not owned by the publisher.

The Hachette Speakers Bureau provides a wide range of authors for speaking events. To find out more, go to hachettespeakersbureau.com or email hachettespeakers@hbgusa.com.

Little, Brown and Company books may be purchased in bulk for business, educational, or promotional use. For information, please contact your local bookseller or the Hachette Book Group Special Markets Department at special.markets@hbgusa.com.

Illustrations by Abby Eblen, MD, MSHS
Print book interior design by Bart Dawson

ISBN 9780316578769
LCCN 2025934257

Printing 1, 2025

LSC-C

Printed in the United States of America

To Rick, Benjamin, and Hailey. You are truly
the reason this book was conceived.
I love you to the moon and back.

To Mark, Ava, and Jack. You are my best.
I love you all the amounts.

To Brook, Beck, Blaine, and Brynn.
Your love and support give me strength,
and your joy inspires me every day. I love you.

You may encounter many defeats, but you must not be defeated.

— Maya Angelou

CONTENTS

· ·

PART III

WHAT HAPPENS AFTER IVF?
Preparing for the Next Chapter

PART IV

UNIQUE FAMILY JOURNEYS
The Evolving Role of IVF

The

I V F

Blueprint

INTRODUCTION

$\cdots\cdots\cdots\cdots\cdots\cdots\cdots\cdots\cdots\cdots\cdots\cdots\cdots$

Reliable and cutting-edge information about IVF (in vitro fertilization) is challenging to find from any source. We want this book to give you both. Thinking about IVF may make you feel hesitant, anxious, or even terrified. However, the more you know about the process, the better you will feel as you go through your IVF journey. If you are thinking about IVF or in the midst of it, this book is for you. We have divided it into four sections to allow you to find your desired information quickly.

So, what is IVF? It is a way to use medication to stimulate the growth of approximately one year's worth of eggs simultaneously, usually around twelve eggs at a time instead of just one. A minor procedure is done to remove the eggs while you are under sedation. In the IVF lab, sperm joins with the eggs to create embryos. Embryos grow in an incubator until they are about five days old.

The growth and development of an embryo is a complex process that is not fully understood. As a result, not all eggs will be fertilized and result in embryos. About one-third to one-half will survive until the fifth day. At that stage, we remove cells from the future placenta to determine if the embryo has the correct genetic material. For healthy women, it is typical to have one to three genetically normal embryos. Usually, one normal embryo is transferred about six weeks later. During that time, you will receive estrogen and progesterone to turn your uterus into a nurturing environment. The medicine will continue throughout the first twelve weeks of pregnancy. At this point, you will stop the medication, and the baby's placenta will provide all the hormones necessary for the remainder of the pregnancy.

We've just described the IVF process in a nutshell. However, there is much more to tell you, and we will go into detail about each aspect. The information in this book will help you get started and have the family of your dreams. But first, let us tell you a little about who we are. We are three board-certified reproductive endocrinology and infertility doctors who walk patients through IVF and perform in vitro fertilization procedures every day. We took three different paths to our current practices, training in three different medical schools, residencies, and fellowships for eleven years after college. We met and began collaborating on a podcast, *Fertility Docs Uncensored,* in 2020. During our interactions with listeners, we received hundreds of questions and uncovered a strong desire to understand more about IVF. For many, confusion occurs because of the voluminous amount of complex information given quickly in the doctor's office. We will review the information you missed when you first heard it, and we'll provide additional details to make your journey less confusing!

We are true insiders, but not just because of our training. It turns out being fertility docs didn't make us immune from infertility ourselves. We understand the anxiety of being an infertility patient and the difficulty of taking the plunge to start IVF. Two of us have been on the other side as IVF patients. Abby became a patient *after* she became a fertility doctor. Here is an excerpt of her story:

> When I finally finished my years of medical training, I was
> ready to be a mom. Every month I tried, I'd get my period,

and as a fertility doctor, I knew exactly what that meant — I wasn't pregnant. Eventually, I had to face the fact that I was part of the one in eight couples with infertility. It felt like being a mechanic who couldn't even fix her own car!

The emotional toll began to weigh on me. I knew it was time to start treatment when tears began to flow during a children's choir performance at church. I wondered if I'd ever be a mom. Although it was tough to admit I needed help, I confided in my colleagues and was comforted by their support.

There were lots of shots, blood draws, and ultrasounds. The shots were daunting for about three days, but soon I accepted I was a human pincushion and began jabbing myself like a pro. All of that poking and probing *every day* was more irritating than I had ever imagined when I was on the other side as the doctor. It made me a little grumpy. Who wouldn't be? Right after my eggs were retrieved, I had more abdominal discomfort than I expected and felt as if I had done a bunch of sit-ups. The pain was gone by the next day. The real nail-biter was waiting to see if I'd actually get pregnant.

My embryo did not excel during the thaw. It was not "pretty" compared to the ones I had seen in the recent past. As a result, I cried through the transfer, my years of training telling me there was no way it would work. But miraculously, that four-cell embryo was meant to be, sent from God. Two years later, I had two more frozen transfers, and the final one resulted in my second baby. This experience taught me to always stay hopeful even when science tells me otherwise. In my case, I learned that miracles do happen, and a sad-looking embryo can still surprise you!

Susan also had her own IVF journey:

My fertility journey started years before I did IVF. Shortly before my husband and I tried to conceive our first child, I was diagnosed with Graves' disease (an autoimmune disease that causes an overactive thyroid). While I was under medical treatment for Graves', we tried to get pregnant for about six months. But, being a little obsessed about things not working quickly and according to my timeline, we decided that my husband would get a semen analysis. He had some serious health issues as a small child, and we both had a lingering concern that those might impact our fertility. Fortunately, the results were normal, and we got pregnant shortly thereafter. I developed severe preeclampsia and delivered preterm. Our second pregnancy, while I was doing my fellowship, followed my diagnosis of celiac disease. We had wanted to conceive sooner, but we needed to make sure that I was healthy. Again, it took us a little over six months until we saw "Pregnant" one morning on the test. This pregnancy was physically harder on me, and I again delivered early due to preterm rupture of membranes.

Some people glow through pregnancy. For me, I survived, and it was a means to a beautiful end. Because of this we were done. I decided to have my tubes tied at the time of my second C-section. A few years later, we got the "baby bug." We talked about our options: do nothing, adopt, tubal reversal, or IVF. For us, IVF was the right decision. When we went through IVF, PGT-A (preimplantation genetic testing for aneuploidy, which we will talk a lot about later in the book) was new. We were working in Texas, but we chose to do IVF on the East Coast at a clinic known for incorporating this technology — not something I would recommend unless there is a very good reason behind it. In my initial workup, it was discovered that I had diminished ovarian reserve (high follicle-stimulating hormone levels and low antral follicle count). Though I knew there were multiple potential contributing factors, including my personal history of multiple autoimmune diseases and possible compromise to the ovarian blood supply at the time of my tubal ligation, it did add another level of stress and personal guilt that I had to navigate.

The logistics of my stimulation, in hindsight, were a bit comical. I did "remote" monitoring at my home clinic in Texas, then flew to my East Coast clinic when I was nearing the end of my stimulation. But my follicles took a while to grow, likely due to my poor ovarian reserve. I remember lining my medications up on the counter of a restaurant in Manhattan to take my injections on an evening when we were trying to do "normal" things. Finally I got triggered and went to retrieval. We got some eggs, but a lower-than-average number from less-than-optimal follicles. Our hopes were tied to those eggs, though, and later to the embryos in the incubator. We returned to Texas for a few days to get back to work, then flew back again for, we hoped, a transfer on day 6. Back then, we thought fresh transfers were always best. I still remember sitting in the hotel restaurant at breakfast and getting the call that we had a chromosomally normal embryo! Fortunately, that precious embryo stuck and developed into our lovely daughter — who rushed into this world a week earlier than her brothers.

We are true insiders, and now you will be too.

Because of our own experience, we want you to be prepared for all phases of the IVF journey. You may want to know what questions to ask your doctor during the initial IVF visit. Some patients want to hear about medications and supplements they can take to give them the best chance of success. Others need to understand how we do an egg retrieval. A few of our patients want to know when they can hit the gym again.

This book is also a good resource for family members who want to understand what you are experiencing — well, maybe not nosy Aunt Betty. It is also a resource for supportive friends, particularly the ones who may be giving you injections. Just make sure they read Chapter 3 before they head toward you with the needle! Others who can benefit from this knowledge are health professionals, new IVF team members, primary care physicians, mental health professionals, and others who work with IVF patients.

Reading the book once or twice (or even ten times) may help the details click into place. There are many details about IVF that you will hear from your doctor and your IVF team. But let's face it, most of us feel like we glaze over after about fifteen minutes of medical information. The volume and complexity can be overwhelming — even for docs! Remembering everything after you have heard it only once is virtually impossible. Hopefully you will use this book as a reference when your brain gets to the information-overload stage.

Our goal is to lift the veil from the IVF journey and make this process more user-friendly. We share all the behind-the-scenes details about the procedures and the inner workings of the embryology lab. This is information most infertility patients want to understand better. We know this because we receive numerous questions about IVF for the "Ask the Docs" segment on our podcast, *Fertility Docs Uncensored*. Now we will get to answer many of those questions with this book. By understanding the process, we hope, you will find IVF a little less daunting. You can do this, and we will walk you through the steps one at a time.

All of your IVF questions will be answered in this book. We know many of you first consult with everybody's friend, Dr. Google. Some of what you read there may be true, but much is not! We want to ensure you get truthful answers to your questions and have a little fun along the way. Altogether, the three of us have been in this field for about fifty years, plus the valuable time we spent as IVF patients!

Some of you may have already met with a reproductive endocrinologist and infertility (REI) specialist — a doctor specializing in the diagnosis and treatment of infertility. If not, that should be one of your next steps. Your infertility team is your best source of fertility knowledge, but time with them is limited. As providers of infertility treatment, we learn from and support each other in our fight against infertility every day. We understand the science of infertility, but there is also an art to the practice of medicine. Because each of us is an individual, we practice the art of medicine in slightly different ways. Many treatments are backed by science, but scientific data is not always available to guide every decision. In those situations, our choice of treatment results from our own unique experiences. If you read this book and your provider does something a little different than the way we discussed, just ask them about it. There is more than one way to accomplish the same result. We hope this will complement what you learn in your doctor's office and give you the confidence to proceed with treatment.

In writing this book, we were guided by questions our podcast listeners wrote about IVF. Those questions elucidated gaps in knowledge about IVF that may be overlooked but are important to you. Our aim is for you to be able to use *The IVF Blueprint* as a handbook through the IVF process. We tried to make the chapters understandable to nonspecialists, whether you read them all the way through or decide to go right to the parts that apply to you.

The book is divided into four parts. The first three cover important information you want to know before, during, and after completing the IVF process. The fourth reviews newer reasons to do IVF. The book is organized chronologically, so you will have easy access to the information you need at every stage of the journey. Along the way, we also include insider tips and tricks that you will find helpful — information that is good to know but probably was not discussed at your IVF consult due to time constraints.

Part I covers what you should consider when preparing for and proceeding with IVF. We discuss IVF medications and the reason you may be taking a specific kind of medication. We mention health issues you may need to "tune up" before starting the journey. We also have a chapter about supplements that might help give your ovaries that extra kick.

Part II discusses information about the stimulation you will undergo before egg retrieval. You will get details about the specifics of the big day, and a behind-the-scenes tour of the egg retrieval process. We share information about the role of team members that you will meet while you are in the surgery center. Embryo development and the kinds of genetic testing you may want to consider are detailed. We will discuss whether doing a fresh or frozen embryo transfer is best.

Part III will cover recovery and embryo transfer. We will discuss how and when you return to normal, possible side effects (including ovarian hyperstimulation syndrome), and when you need to call your doctor if you have symptoms. It provides information about embryo transfer and details of the actual procedure. Finally, we will discuss the monitoring of your growing baby in early pregnancy and when you graduate from us to see your obstetrician.

Part IV discusses other reasons you may want to consider IVF. IVF is no longer done exclusively as a last resort for infertility. It is now done to freeze eggs, to have your female partner participate, or to get help growing your baby with a gestational carrier. It is also done to help improve the odds for women with recurrent pregnancy loss and to prevent you from transferring a genetic abnormality to your baby. We will discuss all of those reasons for IVF in detail. We have not left anything out. This is *the* book you need to read as you embark on IVF. Let us help you in your IVF journey and, most importantly, help you start your family.

NOTE: We embrace the fact that many of our patients choose pronouns and self-identify in the way that feels most comfortable to them. Fertility as a topic is complex and emotional, and this book tries to clarify the process as much as possible. To avoid confusion, we consistently refer to people born with a uterus/tubes/ovaries/eggs as "she/her," "female," and "woman," and people born with a penis/testicles/sperm as "he/him," "male," and "man." The goal is purely to simplify explanations of an overwhelming topic. We know there are many ways to make a family, and we love you for who you are.

PART I

Laying the IVF Groundwork

What to Know Before Treatment Begins

CHAPTER 1

. . . .

What You Need to Know About IVF Before You Start

You wake up, your eyes pop open, and anxiety gnaws in your stomach. Then it hits you: this day is here again. It feels like Groundhog Day, but you think the outcome will be different this time. You crawl out of bed and pee on the test strip. Apprehension turns into fear, and you see an ugly "Negative" result. Tears stream down your cheeks, and sadness turns into anger. You can't keep doing this month after month.

Does this sound like you? Have you considered moving on to in vitro fertilization but are apprehensive? You are not alone. Many couples talk about IVF, think about IVF, and even search the internet to find information about IVF, but then procrastinate. But if you keep putting it off, your chances of success decrease each year. The best time to start is now.

You may feel hesitant for several reasons. Many patients are overwhelmed by the procedures and the injections. Maybe your friend told you IVF drugs made her crazy. Then there are the financial costs and concerns about insurance coverage. You and your partner may not be on the same page about proceeding with treatment, and you fear the physical and emotional toll IVF may take. It can feel like playing the lottery.

However, playing the Powerball lottery would give you a 1 in 298 million chance of winning—that's about a 0.00000335 percent chance of success. By contrast, if you are in your mid-thirties and have never tried to get pregnant, you have about a 15 percent chance of getting pregnant in any given month. If you are infertile and have been having unprotected intercourse for a year, the possibility of pregnancy is 1–2 percent per month. And if you do IVF, you have about a 65 percent chance of success with one try if you genetically test your embryos. Those are some good odds for IVF!

Do You Have to Start with IVF Treatment If You Are Infertile?

No, not necessarily. At the initial visit, you will discuss fertility testing, and after the results of all the tests come back, you'll develop a plan. The thing about fertility testing is that it only touches the tip of the iceberg regarding things that could go wrong during reproduction. Researchers have spent their whole careers trying to decipher the events of the first twenty-four hours after egg and sperm come into contact, and there are still many unanswered questions, which means our tests have limited capabilities. Fertility is complicated. Even if you have all the recommended tests, there is a reasonable chance your doctor won't be able to give you the answer to "Why me?"

Many patients focus on the "why" and can't move on. Our most successful patients keep moving forward. If you are less than thirty-five years old and tests show no apparent reason for infertility, your doctor may recommend treatments that are not as involved or as expensive as IVF. For example, you may want to try therapy with oral medication and intrauterine insemination (IUI) as your initial treatment. IUI is a procedure done in the office in which a provider transfers sperm into your uterus via a syringe and catheter, bypassing some hurdles the sperm would otherwise have to navigate before getting to your egg. We frequently recommend IUI even if your partner's swimmers are less than stellar. The success rate in any given month with oral fertility medications and IUI is about 10 percent. However, if you have monthly cycles, oral medications without IUI are about as successful as having timed sex with your partner, which is what you have already done.

It may be reasonable to start with oral medication and IUI for a few months depending on your testing. But "a few months" generally means no more than four months of treatment. Most successful patients become pregnant in months 1, 2, or 3, and occasionally in month 4.[1] Don't waste valuable time and money with those treatments after the fourth month.

Until recently, fertility docs, including us, offered treatment with fertility injections plus IUI, often after oral medication and IUI had failed. The injectable medication is a synthetic form of a hormone, follicle-stimulating hormone (FSH). It is produced in small quantities from your brain, so you usually stimulate the growth of only one egg each month. We now rarely recommend using that treatment.

The American Society for Reproductive Medicine recently evaluated all available medical studies on infertility treatments.[2] It concluded that a regimen of fertility injections plus IUI is no better than oral medication plus IUI treatment in terms of success. However, the important difference is that fertility injections are more likely to stimulate the release of multiple eggs, which raises the chance of having twins, triplets, or even quadruplets. So there are very few situations in which this course of treatment is now medically indicated.

It's understandable to think that having twins might help you grow your family more quickly, with just one pregnancy. Some couples feel that transferring two embryos may lower the financial burden by reducing the need for an additional cycle. However, this approach can actually lead to greater challenges. Twin pregnancies carry a higher risk of complications such as premature birth, increased time away from work, and the need for advanced medical care. They also bring the financial and emotional demands of caring for two infants at once.[3] According to a study from the American College of Obstetricians and Gynecologists, the cost of raising twins or triplets isn't just double or triple that of a single baby — it can be four to ten times greater. Families of multiples often face added stress, a greater risk of postpartum depression, more strain on relationships, and reduced quality of life. Additionally, research shows that children from multiple births are at increased risk of experiencing abuse.[4] Because of the significant risks and long-term impact on families, we prioritize approaches that help support the healthiest outcomes for both parents and children.

Your doctor may have talked to you about IVF and seemed to be aggressively recommending the most expensive treatment immediately, or after just a few months of other treatment. However, we know what you are about to learn: IVF is the quickest and most successful route to pregnancy. We went into this field because we love helping couples start their families, and IVF gives you the best chance of doing that.

Insider Tips That Will Help You Sail Through Your IVF Journey

The more you know before you start, the easier the journey will be. We want you to have sound and valid information as you start your IVF cycle. So we'll provide helpful tips and tricks to give you the best possible chance of success. For example, some of our patients fear the injections (frankly, no one looks forward to having shots). Some are overwhelmed by the time it takes to complete a cycle. It's true that the road to success can feel like it's winding, complicated, and unending, but it will seem manageable once you have a guide to the IVF blueprint. The tips that we'll provide throughout this book, to help you down the path to your newest family member, include:

1. Understanding the factors to consider before making the IVF leap
2. What questions to ask your doctor at your initial IVF visit
3. Learning how to give yourself the injections
4. Medication side effects
5. Medical conditions needing attention before pregnancy
6. Supplements
7. What we see on vaginal ultrasound
8. Behind-the-scenes details at the egg retrieval
9. IVF terms (such as AMH, ICSI, and PGT)
10. What normal embryo development looks like
11. Deciphering the genetic tests that may be done on your embryos
12. Differences between fresh and frozen transfers
13. A lesson about "the birds and the bees"
14. Returning to normal after the egg retrieval
15. Ovarian hyperstimulation: when to get evaluated
16. Preparation and medications for embryo transfer
17. The connection between pregnancy and hormone levels, and what the numbers mean
18. Third-party reproduction — egg and sperm donation, embryo donation, and gestational carriers
19. LGBTQIA+ family-building
20. Egg freezing to preserve fertility

While IVF can seem overwhelming at first glance, it's important to remember that it's one of the most successful fertility treatments available today. Whether you're still exploring other options or have decided IVF is your next step, knowing what to expect and how to prepare can make a world of difference. By approaching your journey with knowledge, support, and a sense of empowerment, you're already setting yourself up for the best possible experience. IVF isn't just a medical process — it's a path forward, filled with hope, progress, and possibility.

CHAPTER 2

. . . .

Deciding on IVF: The Key Questions and the First Steps

Deciding to do IVF is a big decision you make with both your heart and your head. However, several essential factors involving your personal medical history have a significant impact on your chances of success. After we discuss these topics, you can better discern whether proceeding with IVF is the right decision for you.

A frank discussion with your fertility doctor is essential and helpful. Most people have several fundamental medical, financial, and emotional concerns. Your doctor can address your situation during the consultation and help you decide. Consider these essential factors when trying to determine if IVF is the correct choice for you:

1. Do you have a specific infertility diagnosis, or do you have unexplained infertility?

2. How old are you?
3. Do you have a medical illness that may worsen over time?
4. Can IVF prevent you from having a child with a genetic disorder?
5. Does your insurance cover IVF? If not, can you afford to do it?
6. Are you emotionally exhausted from your fertility journey?
7. Do you need to address religious or ethical beliefs or thoughts prohibiting you from doing IVF?
8. How long have you been trying to get pregnant?
9. Are you unable to carry a pregnancy, need help obtaining eggs or sperm, or want your female partner to participate in the journey?
10. What will happen during the IVF consult?
11. What should I ask my doctor even if I have already asked Dr. Google?

Let's discuss these questions and how they pertain to your decision.

Do You Have a Specific Infertility Diagnosis?

The first step is to undergo fertility tests that should be done before you start the process. These will include, but likely will not be limited to, ovarian reserve testing to determine your egg quality and quantity; a uterine assessment to ensure your embryo has a nice, cozy place to implant; and sperm testing to evaluate the function and number of sperm.

As REI specialists, we do specific tests on almost every patient because those tests give us so much useful information about egg

If you want more information about IVF or infertility in general, go to the website of the American Society for Reproductive Medicine (ASRM). It is a trusted source of fertility information for doctors and patients, providing evidence-based information to guide care.

quantity, uterine and ovarian appearance, sperm quantity, and sperm function. These tests give us a good picture of overall fertility and help determine the best treatment plan.

Let's start with the ovaries and ovarian reserve testing. Females are born with all the eggs we are ever going to get, so we need to make the most of them. Your doctor may want to check your anti-Müllerian hormone (AMH). An AMH level gives us the best idea of how many eggs you have in your ovaries — and more is always better. It can't give us the specific number of eggs left in your ovary. However, based on your AMH level, we can determine if your egg number is appropriate for your age.

An ultrasound evaluation of your eggs can also be valuable in determining ovarian reserve. The number of tiny follicles (those with a diameter under 10 mm; these are often called antral or micro follicles) in your ovary is counted, and that number gives us an estimate of your overall ovarian reserve. Having many small follicles in your ovary suggests you have an even larger pool of follicles that we cannot see. Like an AMH level, measuring antral follicles gives us a gauge of egg quantity. Meanwhile, measuring reproductive hormones secreted from the brain and the ovary — FSH, LH, and estrogen — provides insight into egg quality. (These are sometimes referred to as day 3 hormones, since the best time to check these levels is on the second or third day of the menstrual cycle; levels can vary depending upon when in your cycle we check them.) High levels of FSH (over 10 mIU/ml) by the fourth day of your cycle are abnormal, suggesting your egg quality is poor. We also want to know how much estrogen you're making in response to other hormones; low levels can be expected early in the cycle but should rise and peak midcycle. High estradiol levels early in the cycle may suppress your FSH level and may indicate a functional ovarian cyst or even premature follicular development.

We don't want to leave your male partner out, either. The semen tests you can order on the internet or buy at the pharmacy are not adequate. It is best to go to the experts at your fertility clinic to have a semen analysis done. Fertility clinics do these every day and can give you essential information about your results. More importantly, they can let you know if some of the values listed are concerning — there are many categories to assess, and not all are equally important.

The SpermQT test determines if the sperm has what it takes to bind to and penetrate the egg. For some couples, learning that the sperm is unlikely to break through the outer layer of the egg may help them decide quickly that IVF is a better option for them than IUI.

Making sure your baby has a nice place to live for nine months is a top priority! To do that, we evaluate the inside of your uterus and fallopian tubes before you get pregnant. We can do this non-surgically with a hysterosalpingogram (HSG) or saline ultrasound. We want to ensure you are not pregnant at the time of the procedure. Schedule this early in your menstrual cycle, between days 5 and 11 (the first day of full flow counts as day 1). If you are unable to do the test during this window, you may be asked to start birth control pills to keep your uterine lining (endometrium) thin until the time of your evaluation.

An HSG is the best way to evaluate the fallopian tubes and gives some information about the endometrium as well. A radiologist usually does this test as an outpatient procedure. You are awake during the process. The radiologist will put radiopaque dye inside your uterus slowly, and the dye will fill your uterus and go through your fallopian tubes. Once the dye has spread, X-rays are taken. It is a quick procedure, over within about five minutes. You may have abdominal aching, similar to bad menstrual cramps, for about fifteen minutes afterward, so it is wise to take ibuprofen, if you can, about thirty to sixty minutes before the procedure starts. Most people can drive themselves home. With this procedure, there is a small risk (about 1 percent) of uterine infection, as common germs in the vagina can sometimes get into the uterus as the dye flushes into your reproductive tract. Given the small risk, taking antibiotics before the procedure is necessary only if you are at high risk for a pelvic infection. You should talk to your doctor about the need for prophylactic antibiotics.

Your doctor may also evaluate the uterus with a saline sonogram. It is similar to the HSG but is done under ultrasound. This procedure gives us a better view of the inside of your endometrial cavity. Sometimes air bubbles or radiopaque foam is used during the procedure to help determine if your fallopian tubes are open. Some physicians prefer a saline sonogram before IVF because it provides a better view of the uterine cavity than an HSG.

When your doctor is evaluating the fallopian tubes prior to IVF, the biggest issue is whether you have a hydrosalpinx (swollen tube). The fluid that collects in a hydrosalpinx can be toxic to the embryo and decreases IVF success rates by up to 50 percent. If you do have a hydrosalpinx (or hydrosalpinges in both tubes), it is strongly advised that you have a laparoscopy and have your tube or tubes removed or ligated (blocked). You don't need the surgery before egg retrieval, but it should be done before embryo transfer. Many IVF centers will not permit or strongly caution against an embryo transfer in the presence of a hydrosalpinx.

If a saline sonogram or HSG shows an abnormality within the

uterine cavity, then a hysteroscopy is performed. (However, some physicians prefer to go straight to hysteroscopy in patients who are doing IVF.) Hysteroscopy is an outpatient surgical procedure. No incisions are made; a small, narrow scope is placed inside the uterine cavity to evaluate any abnormalities seen during the initial testing. Other instruments are placed through the scope to remove polyps, fibroids, or adhesions.

You may hear that you have a uterine septum. A uterine septum is a congenital malformation of the uterus — it's the way you were born. When you were a fetus, your uterus started as two separate pieces. Those pieces had to come together and fuse, and the inside had to dissolve. It's a complicated process, so it doesn't happen correctly in everyone. With a septum, the outside of the uterus generally is rounded but the inside of the uterus is divided by fibrous tissue that doesn't have the same healthy blood supply as the rest of the uterus. The septum can be partial, making the uterus heart-shaped, or complete, dividing the uterus into two small spaces instead of one big one. Some docs may remove a partial septum prior to embryo transfer, and most will remove a complete septum; this can be done with tiny scissors inserted through the scope during hysteroscopy.

Any tissue taken from the uterus during hysteroscopy for further examination is usually either a polyp or a fibroid and is rarely dangerously abnormal. Polyps look like skin tags and tend to be soft and squishy. Anyone can get polyps, but those who are at the most risk are overweight, have irregular periods, or have a history of polyps. Polyps are benign (not cancerous) 99 percent of the time in premenopausal women.[1] Even if the analysis shows irregular or precancerous cells, most women can be effectively treated, at least in the short term, with extended exposure to progestins.

Fibroids are firm, like the inside of a tennis ball. They can also be challenging to remove entirely and may require more than one hysteroscopy. The location of the fibroids is important. Fibroids attached to the exterior of the uterus (serosal fibroids) and fibroids within the muscle of the uterus that do not interfere with the endometrium (myometrial fibroids) do not usually pose a significant risk to pregnancy. But fibroids that are partially or completely within the lining of the uterus (submucosal fibroids) or that are very large can interfere with pregnancy success and should be surgically removed before embryo transfer.

Sometimes the tissue removed is lumpy but is not a polyp or fibroid. It doesn't matter — if it is lumpy or bumpy, we want it gone! The benefit of removing this tissue is that it decreases the chances of having what's known as a sterile inflammatory reaction inside the uterine cavity. This inflammatory reaction makes it less likely that the embryo will nestle into your uterine cavity.

Adhesions are the rarest of the abnormalities. Intrauterine adhesions usually result after procedures like D&Cs, which are used to treat a miscarriage or retained placenta, to treat heavy bleeding or abnormalities of the endometrium like hyperplasia or endometrial cancer, or to do an elective termination. Adhesions can also occur with certain systemic illnesses such as tuberculosis or when an infection complicates a uterine procedure (especially a D&C).

Adhesions are scar tissue.

The recovery after hysteroscopic surgery is usually less than twenty-four hours, with minimal postoperative pain. Most people go back to work the following day. This procedure rarely causes a significant delay in proceeding to IVF. Hopefully, your embryo will love your inviting uterine cavity!

Making the Decision

One of the most important deciding factors for IVF treatment is whether you have a specific infertility diagnosis or unexplained infertility. The decision about whether to choose IVF is rarely clear-cut; however, two medical conditions strongly suggest that IVF is the best approach. The first reason to do IVF is to overcome a significantly low sperm count (the medical term for this is "severe oligospermia"). If your partner has a moderately low sperm count, you may want to try less aggressive treatments first, such as IUI (discussed in Chapter 1). But if your partner has a truly meager sperm count or has significant abnormalities in terms of volume or motility, IVF is the best option to get his little guys in your egg.

Most fertility doctors recommend IVF when there is a low amount of moving sperm. To fertilize the egg, a certain number of sperm need to be present and fighting together to make an opening in the egg's outer layer, the zona pellucida. The total number of moving sperm is assessed by calculating the total motile sperm count (determined by multiplying the semen volume by the concentration by the motility). Remember that, as with other measurements, the total motile sperm count will not be the same each time it's tested, but it should be similar. If the total motile count is less than 5–10 million, IVF is the best way to get sperm inside the egg — specifically with a procedure called intracytoplasmic sperm injection (ICSI). During the ICSI procedure, a needle is used to inject sperm inside the egg.

During IVF, the embryologist (the person who grows your embryos) may perform ICSI. If you have ten eggs, the embryologist needs ten sperm, not 10 million. The fertilization rate is about 70 percent using ICSI, but it can vary widely in individual cases based on sperm quality.[21] The other way for fertilization to occur is conventional insemination. With this fertilization procedure, the egg floats near the sperm in a petri dish, and the sperm enters the egg without outside help.

The other medical condition that makes it necessary to do IVF is having two blocked fallopian tubes. You can still get pregnant without IVF if you have one open tube. Fallopian tubes are like kidneys; it is great to have two, but you need only one. However, if you do not have open tubes, it is like driving your car into a blocked tunnel: your car can't make it through. Similarly, sperm can't make it through a blocked fallopian tube. IVF allows us to gather your eggs and your partner's sperm and bypass blocked tubes. In unassisted conception, the magic of fertilization happens in the fallopian tubes. With IVF, it happens in the lab.

But suppose we don't know why you are not getting pregnant. This is unexplained infertility. There is no hard and fast rule about when to do IVF. Generally, if you are under thirty-five and have not used birth control for a year, you may want to try less expensive treatments first, such as the use of oral fertility medication and insemination. During insemination, sperm is placed in your uterus when you are about to release an egg. It is okay to try those treatments for a few months, but don't spend years on them.

How Old Are You?

Your eggs have a shelf life, just like the ones in your refrigerator. Fortunately, the shelf life of your eggs is decades, not weeks. Still, if there is a glitch in our female system, this is it. Women get one set of eggs at birth. Males make new sperm continually over a lifetime. So unfair!

Here is the reality check. No matter how much you exercise, how well you eat, how well you _____ (fill in the blank), your age matters. There are two sets of chromosomes in your eggs. When an egg wakes up each month at ovulation, it must undergo meiosis — that is, it must evict half of its existing chromosomes to make way for the chromosomes provided by the sperm. Sometimes, though, the number of chromosomes it evicts is more or less than half. By the time you're thirty-five, at least half of the eggs you ovulate carry the wrong number of chromosomes. And by the time you're forty, most of your eggs have too few or too many chromosomes. If a sperm fertilizes them, they will not produce a healthy embryo. These unhealthy embryos usually do not result in pregnancy, or if a pregnancy begins, it ends in miscarriage. A small percentage result in a live birth with a chromosomal abnormality like Down syndrome (trisomy 21). The other factor at work is that as you age your egg pool decreases in size, which does not improve your baby-making odds either. Add to that the fact that the ones left behind are not as good as the ones you ovulated in your twenties, and you can see the problem.

The only thing that can help is a treatment that does not take a long time — and voilà, IVF. When you do IVF, we try to get your body to make a year's worth of eggs at one time. We cannot change the quality or quantity of your eggs. However, if you do IVF, you may produce several eggs at once that otherwise would have died. We hope at least one "golden egg" can make a baby. Therefore, your age is one of *the* most important factors to consider.

Do You Have a Medical Illness That May Worsen Over Time?

Perhaps you have a gynecological illness that may worsen over time, and the only definitive treatment is hysterectomy (removal of the uterus) or oophorectomy (removal of ovaries). For example, maybe you have such bad pelvic pain that you can't imagine that people have sex for fun. Your period may be so heavy you take an overnight bag full of pads and a change of clothes to work when your period starts. Perhaps during your cycle, you curl up in a fetal position for a few days popping ibuprofen like Halloween candy. Many people with these symptoms have severe endometriosis, and the only permanent solution for that condition is removing your ovaries. Or you have a precancerous condition in your ovaries, uterus, or cervix, and it's important not to wait so long it turns into cancer. These might be extreme examples, but you get our point: such situations have to be dealt with sooner rather than later. So if you have one of these conditions, the sooner you get pregnant, the better the chances of pregnancy success. And then you can get the treatment you need.

Other health issues can worsen over time, making it better to have children sooner rather than later. For example, autoimmune conditions like multiple sclerosis, ulcerative colitis, lupus, and rheumatoid arthritis fall into this category. Most patients who conceive with these conditions do very well, but the sooner you get pregnant and the younger you are, the more likely it is you will have an uneventful pregnancy. Complicated medical conditions are less problematic if you are under thirty-five and otherwise healthy.

Can IVF Prevent You from Having a Child with a Genetic Disorder?

IVF is not just for infertile women. IVF is the only way to find out if your embryo has the right amount of genetic material before it implants. When sperm and egg join, we can test the number of chromosomes in each embryo and determine which embryos have the right amount. This process is called preimplantation genetic testing for aneuploidy (PGT-A). With this information, we can choose the best embryo, giving you the best chance of conception. Sometimes, genetically testing embryos helps to improve outcomes for women with recurrent pregnancy loss. Each person should have 46 chromosomes inside every cell in the body (see Chapter 11). About 50 percent of miscarriages are due to the wrong number of chromosomes, either too few or too many. By testing the embryos and transferring a genetically normal one, there is a significant decrease in pregnancy loss. Also, doing IVF gives us more control over more steps in the process of conception, and we can create an environment that's more conducive to implantation and pregnancy.

Another benefit of doing IVF with genetic testing of embryos is that couples who carry genetic traits that can lead to significant diseases minimize the risk of passing them to their children when they do IVF with prcimplantation genetic testing for monogenic disorders (PGT-M). Many genetic conditions can cause significant disease or disability in children, including cystic fibrosis, sickle cell anemia, and spinal muscular atrophy, just to name a few common ones. Once we determine whether either partner has one of these genetic abnormalities, probes find the abnormal genes in each embryo through PGT-M. We will only transfer an embryo that either is not affected or, for conditions that emerge only when the embryo receives an abnormal gene from both parents, is only a

Try to find out as much information as possible about your insurance coverage before your first visit. Otherwise, you may hesitate to get recommended labs and ultrasounds done at the initial visit. Your doctor's office can help you with that, but it is unlikely they can provide immediate information about your plan while you are there. Many insurance plans will cover diagnostic testing, ultrasounds, and lab work. Some insurance plans will cover treatment, and others will not. In the past several years, many large employers have begun to provide insurance coverage for IVF. Often they don't publicize fertility coverage, so it is helpful if you ask.

carrier (with one normal copy of the gene and one abnormal copy; the normal copy provides the correct genetic information and prevents the child from having the condition).

Does Your Insurance Cover IVF?
If Not, Can You Afford to Do It?

IVF is indeed expensive. High IVF costs are due to pricey medications, multiple office visits, lab tests, surgery, and babysitting your little ones in the IVF lab. If you have insurance coverage for IVF, insurance often pays for office visits, labs, and surgery; however, plans even from the same employer may be a little different. Find out as much as you can about your specific plan before treatment begins. Most IVF practices will help you determine what is included in your benefits package. While IVF is expensive, as are other medical procedures, the more significant issue is that many employers do not want to provide the insurance coverage that pays for it.

That trend is changing, and many companies are starting to cover infertility testing and treatment. They see how important coverage is to their younger employees and how it helps with employee retention. If you have yet to check with your HR department, you should do that soon. Some companies do not publicize changes in fertility coverage. If you do not have coverage, talk to HR and ask them why not. Many of our patients have been the spark that brought about change at their company.

There are also third parties that provide guarantee programs. One example of that program would be paying for three IVF cycles and getting money back if you are unsuccessful after the third treatment. If you conceive in the first two treatments but you paid for three, they keep all the money you paid initially. Most guarantee programs make you meet specific criteria before they let you participate. As you would expect, the requirements favor young women with a good egg count, since those women are likely to conceive quickly.

Unfortunately, you may need to take out a loan — not unlike when you want to buy a car. However, there are loan companies that specialize in funding fertility care. You will have to decide if your fertility journey is worth the price. There are also organizations that provide grants for some or all of the fertility costs. Each organization will have specific criteria. Often they ask applicants for information about their journey to help decide on recipients. Spending extra time to explain why you are the best recipient may pay off in the long run.

Are You Emotionally Exhausted from Your Fertility Journey?

The most critical question for some couples is whether the gamble of IVF is worth the risk. Do you have the mental endurance to complete this complicated treatment? A study showed that patients with infertility have about the same level of stress as women who are diagnosed with recurrent cancer.[3] Infertility is *draining,* and so is IVF. It is an emotional roller coaster that no one can understand unless they have gone through it. Before going to a fertility doctor, you probably did ovulation predictor kits and timed sex during your fertile window. Then, when your emotional tank was about three-quarters full, you began discussing the issue with your OB/GYN and started fertility medication. After that disappointing three months (or six, nine, or twelve months) of treatment, you made your way to a fertility clinic, using up another quarter of a tank.

When you got to the fertility clinic, you may have felt more upbeat and inspired — at least for a little while. For some people, that is not the case, and emotional energy wanes faster with more months of disappointing news. The question at this point is, how much emotional gas do you have left?

Whether you are in your twenties, thirties, or forties, this question is an important one to ask yourself. IVF is the most aggressive and successful way to get pregnant — it is not guaranteed, but it will give you a much better chance of getting pregnant than anything else you have done. IVF requires a profound commitment and significant emotional strength. If you can dig down deep and take the plunge, though, there is a good chance you will be successful.

Do You Need to Address Religious or Ethical Beliefs or Thoughts Prohibiting You from Doing IVF?

The answer to this is as unique as you are. IVF began more than forty years ago. Back then, many people thought IVF was immoral. The ethics of society change over time, and moral considerations vary based on individual beliefs. Some religions have changed the restrictive views on reproduction that they once had. Now IVF is much more common, and you likely know several people who have successfully done IVF (most probably wish they had taken the leap sooner). However, each person needs to think about their feelings and be comfortable with whether to proceed with IVF. Talking to your peers with similar religious, ethical, or moral standards can often give you insight into your personal path. You may find that there are more options than you imagined. After all, shouldn't everyone be able to have the option to start a family?

Let your doctor know about your concerns. Often we can think of ways to help you get pregnant while adhering to your beliefs. For example, if you want nature to take its course in the petri dish, you can let your egg choose the sperm that will fertilize it (conventional insemination) rather than letting the embryologist pick it. Are you concerned about having too many embryos frozen? If so, we can limit the number of fertilized eggs to try to create only one or two frozen embryos. Are you okay with freezing embryos, or does that make you uncomfortable? Thawed embryos usually do well and often result in a baby. By freezing embryos, you can use the normal ones created. Are you planning to use every embryo, or would you consider donating or discarding ones that you do not want to use?

You may eventually want to conceive with all your embryos, which is lovely. Still, we want to transfer them only one at a time! Are you comfortable genetically testing embryos for a better chance of successful conception? Are you uneasy about discarding the abnormal ones? If that is the case, then avoid genetic testing. These are questions to think about when considering IVF.

How Long Have You Been Trying to Get Pregnant?

Generally, if you have tried for more than a year and had several unsuccessful treatment cycles, IVF is your best next step. Many people hold on to a belief that there is some other test or treatment that no one has shared with them over their many years of infertility. Things like supplements and acupuncture may be helpful but rarely have dramatic results. Sorry to be the bearer of bad news, but if there were a magic bullet out there, your doctor would have told you about it by now. Don't get us wrong — some people can get pregnant after years of infertility without explanation.

Over the past decade, the tests and treatments that fertility doctors do have changed, since many have proven less helpful than expected. For example, we no longer do the postcoital test, anti-sperm antibody test, or sperm penetration assay because they do not improve success rates. Initially, we recommend less expensive options for most couples but move quickly to IVF if those are unsuccessful.

Are You Unable to Carry a Pregnancy, Need Help Obtaining Eggs or Sperm, or Want Your Female Partner to Participate in the Journey?

Like a jigsaw puzzle with one missing piece, some necessary pregnancy ingredients may be missing, too. You may have had your uterus removed due to a medical condition but still have your ovaries. In a rarer situation, you may have been born without a uterus (known as Müllerian agenesis). Both are upsetting if you want to have a baby. However, the good news is that you still have two beautiful ovaries. That means you can go through the IVF stimulation, do egg retrieval, and create embryos. Even though you do not have a menstrual cycle every month, your body still ovulates and produces hormones necessary to ovulate. You likely have many healthy eggs. All you will need is someone to carry the pregnancy — a gestational carrier.

Many male couples want to be parents, too. In that situation, sperm from one or both partners fertilizes a donor's eggs, and their embryo is implanted into a carrier. You will hear more about that in Part IV.

Even if you have all the parts you need, including a uterus, you may want to share this experience with your female partner. We call this process reciprocal IVF. One partner receives medicine to stimulate eggs in the ovary. Once the eggs are retrieved, they are fertilized with donated sperm and placed in the other partner's uterus. It is a nice way to share the experience.

What Will Happen During the IVF Consult?

There is much information to discuss, and you may have many questions. The next step is to schedule a visit with your fertility doctor. So, let's discuss what happens during the IVF consult.

It's okay to seek out information before you discuss IVF with your doctor. We hope this book will be a good resource for you. If you go online for information, ensure the sites you visit are reliable and provide truthful information. We like patients to educate themselves about fertility. However, presenting your doctor with reams of paper to prove that your research has unearthed the cure for your infertility might not be helpful and may waste time. We don't mind discussing studies with you, just not twenty or thirty.

While doing your research, remember that not all studies are conclusive. A poorly designed study that includes only five people will not sway anybody's opinion. It is like flipping five coins and coming up with all heads — the likelihood of that being anything other than chance is very small. If a breakthrough study will significantly impact your care, your doctor probably knows about it. Instead, let your doctor spend time in the consultation sharing the expertise that has taken years to acquire. After all, that is why you came to see an REI specialist.

The questions you ask depend on whether this is an entirely new discussion for you or whether you have already talked to friends or family who have done IVF. They will also depend on whether you are new to fertility care or whether this is the next step of your treatment journey. Each doc has a different style, but there are essential parts of the discussion that all IVF consults share.

In the United States, fertility clinics are required to report annual IVF cycle data, including IVF success rates. The information is sent to the Society for Assisted Reproductive Technologies (SART), and the data is available for review on their website. Often, results are delayed by a couple of years because data about birth outcomes must be collected. The site also has an IVF success estimator. After you answer a few questions, it gives you specific information about your chances of having a baby after an egg retrieval. The site is at sartcorsonline.com.

During your visit, your physician should give you an overview of the process and go into more detail once you and your partner understand the big picture. If you are lost, ask for clarification — it only gets more complicated. Most initial IVF consultations will include the following information:

- A realistic time frame
- Discussion of the number of IVF monitoring visits
- Information about the essential IVF medications
- Description of the egg retrieval
- Information about embryo development and expectations for the final embryo number
- Genetic testing options
- Description of the frozen embryo transfer
- General thoughts regarding the outcome

During your visit, you'll learn about your physician's expectations for the final outcome. These are based on your physician's experience and training, but remember, no one has a crystal ball, so it is an educated guess. If you are young and healthy, you may have ten to fifteen eggs after retrieval but only two or three genetically normal embryos. Many eggs retrieved will not be fertilized or continue to grow beyond the first day. Some patients are sad when they don't end up with as many healthy embryos as they expected, but knowing what reproduction involves may at least prevent you from being surprised. Unfortunately, most of your eggs (and sperm, too) don't have what it takes to get to the finish line.

WHAT TRAINING DID YOUR DOCTORS GET?

- An OB/GYN has four years of college, four years of medical school, and four years of OB/GYN residency, and must pass oral and written board exams.
- An REI specialist must, in addition to the above, go through three years of fellowship training, pass oral and written board exams in reproductive endocrinology and infertility, and commit to ongoing continuing medical education.

What Should I Ask My Doctor Even If I Have Already Asked Dr. Google?

When you go for your IVF consult, here are some things you may want to be familiar with ahead of time:

- Brush up on female and male anatomy. We know it sounds a little funny, but many docs throw out anatomical terms right and left, forgetting that you haven't thought about them since high school biology. If you are trying to figure out which part of the anatomy we are talking about, you may miss other, more important pieces of information. When we discuss *tubes,* we mean fallopian tubes, which are tunnels that allow the sperm to swim to the egg. We may talk about *ovaries,* which contain your eggs. The *cervix* is a structure that connects the uterus with the vagina, like a cork, and it has a small opening, the *cervical canal.* We discuss male plumbing too. *Testes* in a male partner are contained in the *scrotum.* The testes contain *sperm.* Occasionally we mention the *vas deferens,* which transports sperm from the testes; part of the vas deferens is removed if a vasectomy is performed, so this is often mentioned if a male patient has had a vasectomy but now wants to father another child. An *embryo* is a fertilized egg, and a *blastocyst* is an embryo that has grown in the IVF lab for five to seven days.

- Genetics is complex for both the doc explaining it and the patient hearing about it. Everyone's knowledge is at a different level, and understanding basic information will make you feel less overwhelmed. Knowing we all have 23 *pairs* of chromosomes (46 total) is helpful, and that a chromosome looks like a big *X.* Half of your chromosomes (23) are from your mom, and the other half (23) are from your dad. If your embryo has too few or too many chromosomes, it is unlikely that successful conception will occur. If you do conceive, you will either have a miscarriage or deliver a living child who will be genetically abnormal.

Genes are small pieces of chromosomes. This is a very important distinction. We often test embryos with PGT-A to see if they have too few or too many chromosomes. Sometimes we also go a step further and test for gene abnormalities with PGT-M. In order to determine if your embryo needs to be tested for an abnormal gene, we have to test you and your partner first. If both of you carry a gene associated with a recessive disorder (diseases such as cystic fibrosis, mentioned earlier in this chapter, that affect a child only if the child inherits two copies of an abnormal gene, one from each parent), or if one of you carries a dominant condition, you should also consider doing PGT-M.

Practical Tips You Should Know
Before Your Consult

- Make sure you are on time for the appointment — you do not want to get the abbreviated version of a thirty-minute consult in fifteen minutes. Make sure you are well rested. Eat breakfast if the appointment is in the morning, and bring a snack if the visit is close to lunchtime. There will be much to cover, so minimize distractions from work texts or emails. It is wise to bring records from previous physicians if this is your first visit with your fertility doctor. It is even better to send records ahead of time and make sure they arrive. Record transfer can be arduous; often, a critical piece of information does not make it to the office before your IVF consult, and this causes frustration before the consult even begins.
- Give your doctor your full attention. It is likely they will cover all your questions by the end of the visit, since they often do several IVF consults each day. It is fine to take notes, but you may miss important concepts if you try to get every detail transcribed. Have all your questions written down, since you may feel overwhelmed when your doctor finally wraps up, and ensure they are covered before you leave. You may get printed information about IVF sent to you and even videos about how to do injections. In addition, an IVF nurse will be available during your IVF cycle to answer specific questions as they arise.

- Most patients want to start IVF as quickly as possible. We doctors assume that and try to get the necessary preliminary steps done rapidly. However, you and your partner, male or female, will need testing first. The specific tests required will vary from clinic to clinic, but generally you need bloodwork. Often the female partner needs an evaluation of the uterus, which can be scheduled only for the week after the menstrual cycle. Men need a semen analysis, and the clinic may require an additional frozen sperm specimen for backup. Your doctor may ask you to see a high-risk obstetrician or primary care doctor if you have certain medical conditions that impact pregnancy.
- Before you leave the office, know what your next step should be. Know if you need to initiate it or if the clinic initiates it. If the latter, get an estimate of the time frame in case there is a miscommunication.

With all the stress and anxiety of infertility, it becomes difficult to think logically about proceeding to the next step. IVF is a *huge* step for most people, impacting many aspects of life — physical, emotional, and financial. The questions and tips in this chapter should help you think logically about IVF to make sure it is the right choice for you.

CHAPTER 3

. . . .

Will the Stimulation Meds
Make Me Crazy?

A re you worried that IVF medications might make you "crazy," because that's something you've heard or read about? It's a great question and the one we get most often. And the answer is probably not! The medications commonly used in an IVF cycle are usually tolerated very well. In this chapter, we will dive into the what, when, and why to understand how these medications work to get the eggs and the ovaries ready for egg retrieval. The medications needed for frozen embryo transfers will be reviewed in Chapter 13.

As we discuss different medications and their typical uses, please remember there is an art to ART (assisted reproductive technology). Your physician's experience is invaluable when creating a customized plan for you. We want you to feel comfortable with the plan and understand the path for your fertility journey. If you are uncertain why your physician chose a specific regimen, please ask!

When we talk about IVF medications, it is easiest to group them into four categories: preparation meds, stimulation meds, ovulation preventers, and triggers. Most of these medications are

Helpful hint: Icing the area or applying a numbing patch before you give yourself the shot really helps, as does massaging the area after the injection! And have your clinic nurses draw circles on your butt or belly in marker to help guide you to potential injection sites.

administered as subcutaneous injections, just barely under the skin, and these injections are usually given with a very thin, short needle. Your nursing team will teach you how to do these injections, and most people can administer the shots themselves.

Anticipation of that first dose is the worst, but once you get past it, you will find the shots aren't that bad. If you have some intramuscular injections, which go deeper, into a muscle, and use a longer needle, you will likely need your partner or a friend to help — it is tough, though not impossible, to do those yourself!

Of note, the medications we discuss here are the most popular in the United States. If you are outside the United States, the brand names may be different.

BUT FIRST, THE BASICS

To truly understand the goal of the medications, you need to know how babies are made.

The vast majority of eggs are stored deep within the ovary and do not respond to hormonal stimulation. Each month, a small group of those eggs, typically between ten and twenty, comes out of storage and begins to grow in response to various hormonal signals from the brain, ultimately leading to ovulation or the release of the egg.

At the beginning of your menstrual cycle, a gland in the brain called the hypothalamus produces a hormone called gonadotropin-releasing hormone (GnRH). GnRH releases impulses that stimulate the pituitary (another gland in the brain) to produce follicle-stimulating hormone (FSH) and luteinizing hormone (LH). The pituitary releases FSH and low levels of LH to signal the ovaries to grow an ovarian follicle, the house of an egg. These hormones support follicle growth and egg development. Estrogen levels increase as the follicles with their supporting granulosa cells multiply and grow. In a normal ovulatory cycle, levels of estrogen increase slowly. When the brain registers this slow increase, while estrogen is still at a relatively low level, it slows the production of LH and FSH. This permits only the strongest of the follicles to survive and keep growing. Usually, only one follicle out of any given month's group grows significantly; all the others in that group die off because they don't have enough support.

Follicles are fluid-filled sacs surrounding the egg.

The subsequent drastic rise in estrogen from this single, dominant follicle sends a signal back to the pituitary, which then quickly and substantially increases levels of LH. That spike in LH, the LH surge, leads to egg maturation and ovulation, or release of the egg. Ovulation predictor kits detect this LH surge.

Stimulation medications given in an IVF cycle mimic these hormonal changes and provide additional support for the growth of all available eggs rather than just one. Other meds prevent egg maturation and ovulation until the moment of readiness, at which point a different medication triggers the maturation and release of the eggs. IVF medications take the elegance of the body's hormonal controls and manipulate them to optimize the opportunity for pregnancy.

The **LH surge** serves as an eviction notice to the eggs. It tells them to grow up and get out of the ovary, beginning their trip down the fallopian tubes to encounter sperm.

Here is a list of the drugs that will be mentioned in this chapter, along with a short description. You may want to refer back to this list as you read through the chapter to help keep the drugs and their uses straight. Notice that leuprolide (which you will often hear referred to by its trade name, Lupron) can be used in several ways depending on its dose and when it is given in the cycle. Therefore, we will distinguish among the uses of leuprolide with the following labels: day 21 leuprolide, microdose leuprolide/leuprolide flare, and leuprolide trigger. Each refers to the same drug, but the purposes are different.

IVF DRUG LIST

THE PREP

- *Oral contraceptive pills.* Help sync the eggs, so they grow as a group.
- *Day 21 leuprolide.* A GnRH agonist taken daily. Helps prevent ovulation later in the cycle as the follicles enlarge.
- *Estrogen.* Helps sync the eggs, so they grow as a group. Estrogen priming is most frequently used in women with decreased ovarian reserve.
- *GnRH antagonist (elagolix [Orilissa] or ganirelix or Cetrotide [cetrorelix]).* Helps quiet the ovaries before stimulation. May be given with estrogen priming.

STIMULATION MEDICATIONS

- *Follitropin-alfa (Gonal-f).* Pure recombinant FSH.
- *Follitropin-beta (Follistim).* Pure recombinant FSH.
- *Menotropin (Menopur).* Purified human menopausal gonadotropin, which provides equal amounts of FSH and hCG-driven LH activity.

Recombinant means human-made using DNA technology to closely mimic the natural hormone structure.

- *Microdose leuprolide.* A specific concentration that, when given at the start of the cycle, causes FSH from the pituitary to "flare." It is given to women with decreased ovarian reserve.

- *Clomiphene citrate (Clomid).* Blocks estrogen receptors and increases FSH levels.
- *Letrozole (Femara).* Lowers estrogen and, in turn, increases FSH levels.

OVULATION SUPPRESSORS

- *GnRH antagonist (elagolix [Orilissa] or ganirelix or Cetrotide [cetrorelix]).* Started when estrogen levels increase and follicles increase in size.
- *Medroxyprogesterone acetate (Provera).* Started at the beginning of the cycle.
- *Day 21 leuprolide.* Started in the previous cycle on day 21, but its purpose is to suppress ovulation.

TRIGGER MEDICATIONS

- *hCG (Pregnyl, Novarel, Ovidrel).* This medication, when given as the final injection in your stimulation, mimics the action of LH, causing ovulation to occur at a certain time.
- *Leuprolide trigger.* When given as the final injection in your stimulation, this formulation causes the pituitary to release LH, causing hormonal changes that lead to ovulation at a particular time. It dramatically decreases your risk of ovarian hyperstimulation.

Now you will learn about each of these medications in detail.

THE PREP

The specific medication that you use before your IVF stimulation varies based on your age, ovarian reserve (how well your ovaries work), and if you have regular monthly periods. If you have a normal ovarian reserve, you often start on oral contraceptive pills (OCPs). Why OCPs? They help the follicles get in sync, so they are all about the same size when the stimulation starts. In IVF, the largest follicles tend to call the shots, so we don't want one racing ahead of the pack and messing up an otherwise tight cohort. Often, fertility patients are not wild about taking OCPs, but remember, they improve your chances of a successful outcome. Common side effects of OCPs are mood swings and intermittent vaginal bleeding or spotting. Most people can tolerate these bothersome side effects for a few weeks, until it's off to the races! After taking OCPs for two to three weeks, you may start another medication, leuprolide, starting on day 21 of your previous cycle, at a dose that prevents premature ovulation later in the cycle (we call this day 21 leuprolide). Other protocols require you to stop the OCPs and go straight into the stimulation meds (gonadotropins).

If you have low ovarian reserve or are older, you may do other types of prep meds. In an estrogen priming cycle, the general premise is giving just enough estrogen to make the brain register a slow increase. This mild increase in levels slows the natural FSH and LH production, preventing follicles from growing prematurely. Like premedication with OCPs, this allows the follicles to get in sync so they are similar in size when stimulation starts. To do this, about a week after ovulation, you start taking estrogen (often in the form of patches or tablets). Another group of medications called GnRH antagonists (discussed later) can be given concurrently. These medications allow the ovaries to rest for about a week before stimulation starts. That way, when stimulation starts, the follicles are ready to party! Another protocol is called a microdose leuprolide flare. Leuprolide starts at the beginning of the stimulation cycle and pumps up the signals to your ovaries to stimulate follicle growth.

STIMULATION MEDICATIONS

The stimulation (stim) medications send signals to the ovaries to start follicle growth, mimicking the action of the pituitary hormones on the ovaries.

Gonadotropins

In the United States, the most common medications include follitropin-alfa (Gonal-f), follitropin-beta (Follistim), and menotropins (Menopur), all given by injection. Follitropin-alfa and follitropin-beta are recombinant forms of FSH (the same hormone the brain produces to stimulate the ovary). Menotropins, purified human menopausal gonadotropin, provide FSH and hCG-driven LH activity. LH and hCG have very similar structures, so they can be used interchangeably. hCG has a much longer half-life compared to LH (meaning it remains in the body longer), thus allowing for once-daily dosing. Most often, follitropin-alfa or follitropin-beta is used either alone or in combination with menotropins. However, some situations (such as hypothalamic amenorrhea) specifically require the exclusive use of menotropins.

The dose of medication will depend on your specific clinical scenario but is often inversely related to your ovarian reserve. For example, a twentysomething with lots of follicles will require much less medication than a forty-year-old with diminished ovarian reserve. Alternatively, some women with severely diminished ovarian reserve may be prescribed a lower dose under certain stimulation protocols because they won't grow many eggs regardless of the dose, so why burn through larger

> **Menotropins** are extracted from the urine of postmenopausal women and then isolated and purified. Fun fact: At first, pharmaceutical researchers worked with retired nuns in Italy to collect large amounts of postmenopausal women's urine at once.

amounts of an expensive medication that won't change the outcome? There are many ways to dose the medications, and if you don't understand why a specific dose was selected for you, ask your doctor. Most people tolerate gonadotropins well and have few side effects when taking them.

Microdose Leuprolide Flare

Here again we encounter the miracle drug leuprolide. As we've seen, its purpose is to control the ovaries. But in a microdose leuprolide flare (unlike day 21 leuprolide, which is given over a longer period to completely shut down stimulatory hormones from the brain to the ovary before gonadotropins are started), the aim is to elicit a small burst of FSH and LH from the pituitary to augment ovarian stimulation. Typically, a microdose leuprolide flare is given if you have a poor response to the average dose of medication. These small doses are given by injection daily with gonadotropins and often decrease the amount of gonadotropin needed to produce follicular growth. You cannot rely on this to produce FSH and LH from the pituitary forever, but it works well for the roughly two weeks it takes to grow mature follicles.

Clomiphene Citrate

Clomiphene citrate (Clomid), given as a pill, is frequently used as a first-line medication to induce follicular recruitment in timed intercourse or intrauterine insemination cycles. Clomiphene belongs to a family of medications called selective estrogen receptor modulators. In the section "But First, the Basics" we discussed how high versus low estrogen levels evoke different responses from the glands in the brain that ultimately impact ovarian function. Clomiphene interferes with estrogen receptors to trick the brain into producing higher levels of FSH, thereby giving an extra bump in FSH level without the need to administer additional injectable medications.

There is a limit to how much FSH clomiphene can elicit, so this is not often used by itself in IVF stim cycles for regular patients, but it is a valuable adjunct.

MINI IVF PROTOCOLS

These protocols use minimal amounts of injectable medications, frequently paired with oral medications such as clomiphene, to achieve follicular growth. These types of cycles are most appropriate for patients who have few follicles or who want only a few eggs. Frequently, multiple cycles are needed to gather enough eggs to create embryos. The decreased cost of meds somewhat offsets the increased expense of multiple retrievals.

Letrozole

Letrozole (Femara) is a similar medication, also given as a pill, often used to recruit follicles to grow during cycles that use timed intercourse or intrauterine insemination. Letrozole belongs to a family of drugs called aromatase inhibitors. Aromatase is an enzyme responsible for converting other hormones to estrogen in the body. In a stim cycle, reducing the activity of aromatase, as letrozole does, often serves to keep estrogen levels low throughout the cycle. This is particularly important for patients with estrogen-sensitive disease, most often breast cancers. This allows us to minimize estrogen exposure while still obtaining as many mature follicles as possible.

OVULATION SUPPRESSORS

Because the goal of IVF is to retrieve several eggs at once, all protocols will use some medication that helps prevent the body from ovulating the eggs too early. The two most common ovulation preventers are GnRH agonists (leuprolide [Lupron]) and GnRH antagonists (ganirelix or Cetrotide). These medications prevent a spike in LH (the LH surge), which leads to ovulation or release of the eggs. In an IVF cycle, we don't want the pituitary to release the eggs too early, which is why ovulation suppressors are used. Communication between the brain and the ovaries must be tightly controlled to keep your eggs in the follicles until egg retrieval.

The first group, GnRH agonists, has already been discussed. They suppress the ovaries before stim and initiate the release of hormones from the pituitary to help activate follicle growth. GnRH agonists attach to receptors on the pituitary and prevent the secretion of the substance that leads to an LH surge. When used this way, GnRH agonists are usually started before the beginning of the cycle (as with day 21 leuprolide), as we reviewed in the section "The Prep." Once any stimulatory effect has passed, the ovaries effectively have no follicular growth yet and are quite receptive to instructions via gonadotropins. Leuprolide stops communication from the pituitary to the ovaries and prevents an LH surge from occurring without your doctor's "permission." The amount given depends on the protocol determined by your physician, as dose and timing critically influence what type of effect leuprolide will have. This class of medications is very effective. However, if your protocol calls for using GnRH agonists to prevent ovulation, they cannot also be used as a trigger — we cannot use them both ways in the same cycle. Most patients tolerate low doses of GnRH agonists well, and the most common side effect is hot flashes.

The second group, GnRH antagonists are often started about a third of the way through stimulation, depending on follicle size and estrogen levels. Commonly these medications are started when follicles are around 14 mm in diameter or when the patient has an estrogen level over 400 pg/mL. Few side effects are usually felt from this group of medications.

The use of antagonists has increased in popularity because they permit the use of leuprolide, hCG, or a combination of the two as a trigger. Patient safety is improved when agonists are used as a trigger.

A new oral form of GnRH agonist, elagolix (Orilissa), may also be used to prevent ovulation. Its timing is the same as GnRH antagonists, rather than the other GnRH agonist we talk about (day 21 leuprolide).

Just as in fashion, what is old can become new again in the fertility world. In the last few years, an oral medication called medroxyprogesterone acetate has found a new role. This medication has historically been used to help women get periods if they have irregular cycles. Now it is more commonly being used throughout a stimulation to prevent premature ovulation, especially in high responders, like egg donors.

TRIGGER MEDICATIONS

Remember the LH surge we mentioned previously, the hormonal event we worked so hard to prevent earlier in the cycle? Well, now we must re-create or provoke it at a very specific time. The LH surge does more than crack open a follicle to release the egg. It also starts a chain of events leading to egg maturation. We want that egg to be mature (not immature or overly mature) at the time of egg retrieval. Only a properly mature egg has the correct machinery and programming to accept a sperm for successful fertilization.

The trigger meds are administered thirty-four to thirty-seven hours before retrieval. Your physician and clinical team will instruct you on the specific time. This is the *most* important medication to administer at a particular time. The timing of the other meds allows for some wiggle room, but your trigger shot does not. *If you take your trigger shot at a different time than instructed, tell your doc immediately.*

Now you know why the trigger shot is so important, but what are the options? Historically, hCG was the medication of choice for the trigger. And if you are using a protocol that utilizes leuprolide to prevent ovulation, such as the long leuprolide protocol, it is still the only option. As we mentioned before, the structure of hCG is very similar to LH, so it makes a very good substitute, especially because LH is hard to "bottle up" for commercial purposes. The body clears (eliminates) a dose of LH within twenty minutes to two hours; this is very quick compared to hCG, which has a clearance time of approximately twenty-four hours. Thus, hCG (sold as Pregnyl, Novarel, and Ovidrel) is a more stable choice to produce the desired result. But that stability and long life in the bloodstream can also have a downside: hCG can overstimulate the ovary past the retrieval, which can tip you into ovarian hyperstimulation syndrome (OHSS) if you're already on the edge, with serious consequences. Chapter 12 will give you the skinny on OHSS.

Leuprolide, which we've encountered before, can serve as a very effective trigger shot. Given in a slightly higher dose, leuprolide stimulates the pituitary to produce an LH surge and then immediately suppresses the hormones that can lead to OHSS, so it can be a safer option for women at high risk. (Sometimes leuprolide and hCG are used together to give an extra little push.) A downside to leuprolide is that it takes the body a while after a dose to build up the stores of pituitary receptors needed for another trigger, which can cause some limitations if you need back-to-back cycles. Another limitation of leuprolide is that it depends on a fully functional pituitary. Patients with certain conditions, such as hypothalamic amenorrhea, may not respond appropriately to the leuprolide trigger and may need hCG instead. Your doctor has carefully selected your trigger meds based on your protocol and ovarian reserve, but if you don't understand the reason for the choice, it's always a good idea to ask.

THE SCARY STUFF, AKA SIDE EFFECTS

While all medications can cause side effects, fortunately the scary ones are quite uncommon. However, we would be remiss not to give you some guidance on what needs immediate medical attention. Regarding your injection sites for gonadotropins, GnRH agonists, or antagonists, it is common to have a local reaction that can look like a small red circle around the injection. This should fade quickly (within thirty to sixty minutes). A local skin reaction, bruising, or irritation is the primary side effect of these injections. Menopur, in particular, occasionally produces a burning sensation. If you have a growing local reaction, any trouble breathing, or swelling of the face, go immediately to your local emergency department.

The most common effect of these medications is they can lead to bloating as your ovaries increase in size. Normal ovaries are the size of a lime, whereas stimulated ovaries can be as large as grapefruits. The end result can make you feel like you have just eaten three large Thanksgiving dinners but have not gone to the bathroom yet. It does not result in pain, but patients are very clearly uncomfortable. This will resolve on its own once you stop medications and get your next period.

Many patients worry about taking "high levels of hormones." These gonadotropins, FSH and LH, prompt the ovaries to grow follicles. If the ovaries do not function, as is the case in postmenopausal women, you could take astronomical amounts of gonadotropins and have absolutely zero response, because the amount of FSH and LH your brain produces during menopause dwarfs any amount you would take during IVF stimulation.

To put into perspective the amount of estradiol and progesterone you may be exposed to during your stimulation cycle, let's talk about what happens in pregnancy. No matter how the baby originates, during pregnancy levels of estrogen and progesterone are ten to 100 times higher than in a normal menstrual cycle and stay elevated for nine months. A stimulation cycle elevates hormone levels, but they are generally truly high for less than a week. While it is always possible to have an adverse reaction (say, a blood clot or stroke in response to elevated estrogen levels), this occurs in well under 1 percent of cases and is far more likely to occur in pregnancy than during an IVF stimulation.

Mindset plays an important role in how patients tolerate these medications. For example, egg donors respond robustly to gonadotropins because they are young with high follicle numbers. Their hormone levels reflect this response. Low-responding patients, whether the low response is due to follicle numbers or to age, tend to experience much lower hormone levels. Egg donors often tolerate these higher levels very well, but their mindset during this experience greatly differs from that of intended parents, those who undergo this process because they want to become parents. Egg donors enter this process as an act of service to build a stranger's family and have the warm and fuzzy feelings associated with that; they still feel the effects of the stimulation, but their mindset helps them tolerate the elevated hormone levels well. People seeking to become parents, on the other hand, enter this process with the weight of the world on their shoulders. If the stimulation doesn't work, it jeopardizes their own dreams of a family. That is far more frightening. As a result, we typically see a more emotional response from intended parents because they have more at stake. Exceptions exist to every rule, but mindset greatly influences a patient's ability to tolerate irritations associated with medication and hormone levels.

The IVF process involves a lot of changing hormone levels. Most women tolerate them well. However, these shifts in hormone levels can pose some risks. As mentioned previously, high hormone levels increase the risk of blood clots. Blood clots can happen anywhere in the body, but the most concerning places include the legs, arms, lungs, and brain. If you have unusual pain in your limbs, chest pain, shortness of breath, or any symptoms of cognitive decline, go to your local emergency department. Leg swelling on just one side also merits evaluation right away. Very rarely, women may experience severe mood disturbances. If you have thoughts of hurting yourself or others, contact medical help immediately. Your safety is the number one priority of your REI specialist; baby-making is number two. However, we can't help you if you don't tell us. If you have a concern, call your physician's office. If it is after hours, there will be an on-call service, so you can talk to a covering physician at your clinic.

. . . .

CHAPTER 4

Getting Ready for IVF:
It's Like Building a House

Often, when faced with IVF, the only thing you can focus on is what is immediately before you: the medications, the appointments, and the procedures. However, it is also important to remember that your physical and mental health are just as critical. A healthy body and mind not only increase the likelihood of IVF being successful but also ensure that both you and your baby have the best chance of a healthy pregnancy and delivery. As REI specialists, we often see people with complex medical histories who are seeking help to conceive. This chapter explores some of the health conditions that can negatively affect pregnancy and what you can do personally and in conjunction with your other physicians to best prepare for IVF and pregnancy and prevent unnecessary delays. To make this big topic a little less overwhelming, we will break things down by organ systems. This is not an exhaustive list, but we do try to touch on the more common maladies.

CIRCULATORY SYSTEM

Okay, let's get to the heart of the matter! Pregnancy and delivery impose the largest strain your heart and your circulatory system will likely ever experience. Changes to the circulatory system during pregnancy are naturally designed to support fetal growth and prepare for the realities of delivery. One such change is an increase in blood volume. The average woman has about 5 liters of blood within her circulatory system. This increases by approximately 50 percent to about 7.5 liters during pregnancy to provide adequate oxygen and nutrients to the developing baby. Since the average delivery results in a blood loss of 0.5 to 1 liter, this extra blood volume serves as a protective mechanism for the mother. To deal with a larger blood volume, the heart increases its workload (cardiac output) by increasing both the amount of blood pumped with each heartbeat as well as the heart rate. Pregnancy hormones relax blood vessels, which decreases systemic vascular resistance (the resistance to blood flow throughout the circulatory system). This increases blood flow to the uterus and placenta to support a growing baby. As the baby grows, the uterus enlarges, which can compress the inferior vena cava, the major vessel in the pelvis responsible for sending blood back to the heart. This can happen in later pregnancy when lying on your back, which can lead to decreased blood pressure and possible fetal heart rate abnormalities (and the associated light-headedness or nausea for mom).

All pregnancies have risks of circulatory system complications, including high blood loss during delivery (hemorrhage), development of blood clots (thromboembolism), dysfunction of the heart muscle (cardiomyopathy), and blood pressure complications (preeclampsia or eclampsia). Though maternal deaths are rare in the United States, they do occur. In 2021, 1,205 maternal deaths were recorded, which is a rate of 33 deaths for every 100,000 deliveries.[1]

Hemorrhage, or high blood loss, accounts for about 12 percent of those deaths.[2] Additionally, pregnancy hormones like estrogen can increase the risk of blood clotting. While such hormones can reduce bleeding at delivery, they also put pregnant women at risk of clots in places we don't want them; the risk can be as high as five times that of someone who is not pregnant, with a rate of 1 to 2 cases out of every 1,000 pregnancies.[3] Blood clots most often originate in the deep veins of the legs, and they can break off and travel to the lungs, leading to a pulmonary embolism. Pulmonary embolisms account for another 10 percent of maternal deaths. Cardiomyopathy is a condition that can arise in women with no history of cardiac disease. The muscle of the heart becomes thickened and enlarged, which limits the heart's ability to effectively pump blood. Cardiomyopathy accounts for about 12 percent of maternal deaths.[4]

Preeclampsia is a medical condition that develops in pregnancy and is characterized by high blood pressure and protein in the urine. There are some risk factors for preeclampsia that can't be avoided; these include a first pregnancy, a first pregnancy with a different male partner, or being pregnant over age thirty-five. However, there are other risk factors that can be modified, such as being overweight (having a high BMI), uncontrolled high blood pressure prior to pregnancy, and the presence of prepregnancy glucose elevation (prediabetes or diabetes). Getting these things in check can make pregnancy and delivery safer and more enjoyable. The severity of preeclampsia can vary from mild to severe, with concurrent liver and kidney dysfunction. Though some treatments are available to help keep a woman and baby safe during labor and delivery, the only true treatment for preeclampsia is delivery. In rare cases, eclampsia may result. Eclampsia is a seizure disorder unique to pregnancy and the early postpartum period (the time just after delivery). The overall mortality rate from eclampsia is about 6.4 per 10,000 cases, with the highest risk when eclampsia occurs before the third trimester.[5]

For these reasons, we need to ensure the cardiovascular system is in good shape. If you were born with a heart defect, especially one that required surgical correction, it is smart to have a cardiology evaluation to make sure all is well. Depending on the nature of the defect, you should be advised if pregnancy poses a significant threat to your health and well-being. The more complex the nature of your heart defect, the more seriously you should consider alternatives such as the use of a gestational carrier.

High Blood Pressure (Hypertension)

It is best to have chronic high blood pressure under optimal control before getting pregnant. The best advice is to work on lifestyle (see Chapter 5) and use medications, if necessary. The most commonly used antihypertensive medications that are safe during pregnancy are alpha-methyldopa, labetalol, and nifedipine. Sometimes you may need to use a combination of medications. ACE inhibitors and diuretics are not recommended during pregnancy. It is wise to be on a favorable medication regimen before conceiving rather than changing once pregnant. Optimizing medications before pregnancy allows for the best control of your high blood pressure. This gives your baby the least risk of exposure to your untreated medical condition or multiple medications.

Pulmonary Hypertension

If you have a certain type of hypertension called pulmonary hypertension, carrying a pregnancy is very risky. This type of high blood pressure results from a dysfunction of the pulmonary artery, the vessel that takes blood from the heart to the lungs. In addition to causing a 25–56 percent maternal mortality rate, severe pulmonary hypertension can decrease blood flow to the placenta, leading to intrauterine growth restriction.[6] Growth restriction can be dangerous for the baby and lead to an increased risk of preterm birth and risks associated with prematurity. These can lead to a more difficult start for a newborn.

Genetic Conditions

Certain inherited or genetic medical conditions such as Turner syndrome (monosomy X) or Marfan syndrome predispose women to a weakening of the structural integrity of the aorta (the main vessel leaving the heart). These abnormalities increase the risk of catastrophic events such as aortic rupture, which is life-threatening to both mother and baby. If you have these conditions, it is important to let your REI specialist know so that appropriate testing and counseling are available to you, and you have the information to make an educated decision about your reproductive future.

Anemia

A common issue for many women, pregnant or not, is anemia (low red blood cell count). As we mentioned earlier, delivery can result in significant blood loss, so if you are starting your journey with a low red blood cell count, it can pose risks to you later. If you have a history of anemia, let your physician know, and they will likely check your CBC (complete blood count) to see if you need help building up your blood supply before pregnancy. Commonly, oral iron supplementation will build up your blood supply to a safe level for you and your baby. In rare cases, women may even need transfusions of blood or IV infusions of iron to help.

> **Iron supplementation** frequently causes constipation. Start a stool softener, extra fiber, or prune juice with it to save yourself the discomfort.

RESPIRATORY SYSTEM

Good oxygenation is important to baby-making. Fortunately, the respiratory system is rather resilient in women of reproductive age. With that being said, the main chronic respiratory issues that impact pregnancy are smoking, asthma, and sleep apnea. Good oxygenation is key for healthy eggs, a healthy mom, and a healthy baby. Managing chronic respiratory conditions is the first step.

Asthma

Asthma is a common chronic respiratory condition, an inflammatory disease that causes increased mucus production and narrowing of the airways. Asthma can vary from mild to severe and can wax and wane during different decades of life. In a woman's reproductive years, asthma is usually at its least bothersome. But asthma symptoms may increase during pregnancy in as many as 5–8 percent of women in developed countries and up to 13 percent worldwide, with more exacerbations in those with more severe asthma at baseline.[7] In addition, things like exercise and respiratory infections can cause asthma exacerbations. If you have asthma, let your physician know. If you require a rescue inhaler (like albuterol) more than two times per week, you should talk to your primary care physician or pulmonologist about additional preventative medications to keep your asthma controlled. Uncontrolled asthma can increase the risk of pregnancy-related complications like preeclampsia, preterm labor, and low birth weight. While undergoing IVF, you will also likely have a form of anesthesia called conscious sedation, where you are ideally breathing on your own but you do not feel or remember anything; having uncontrolled asthma can increase the risks of anesthesia, including aspiration (breathing stomach contents, saliva, or mucus into your respiratory system) or the need for intubation (having a breathing tube placed to support your breathing). Intubation is not a terrible thing, but it can make recovery from egg retrieval slower. Aspiration, on the other hand, can lead to a non-infectious form of pneumonia that can be very dangerous.

Sleep Apnea

Sleep apnea is becoming a common medical condition in the general population. Though mostly diagnosed in older adults, it can also occur in children or young adults. Sleep apnea is a condition in which there can be pauses in breathing or shallow breathing during sleep. This prevents adequate oxygenation, contributing to sleep dysfunction and fatigue, and can make it difficult to manage other chronic conditions (like diabetes, hypertension, or obesity). Sleep apnea can increase complications during IVF anesthesia. During pregnancy, sleep apnea increases the risk of gestational diabetes, preeclampsia, preterm birth, low birth weight, maternal cardiac dysfunction, and abnormal blood clots.[8]

Sleep apnea occurs most often in people who are overweight. However, other factors can play a role, including having a small jaw or a larger neck circumference, smoking or alcohol use, chronic nasal congestion, and a family history of sleep apnea. If you snore, gasp, or choke at night (or have been told by someone else that you do), see your primary care physician to determine if you need a sleep study to assess whether you have sleep apnea. Sleep apnea treatments include weight loss (if weight is a contributing factor) and using a CPAP machine to help keep your airway open while you sleep. These interventions can help you have the best possible pregnancy outcomes.

MUSCULOSKELETAL SYSTEM

Your musculoskeletal system consists of your muscles, bones, joints, tendons, and ligaments. It may not seem that these have much to do with getting pregnant or safely completing a pregnancy. Neverthe-less, issues affecting the musculoskeletal system can impact your chances of a successful pregnancy and delivery.

One of the main hormones of pregnancy is progesterone. In addition to supporting a developing baby, progesterone allows a woman's body to adjust for a growing baby and prepare for deliv-ery. Progesterone relaxes ligaments and tendons. It affects colla-gen, a structural protein, within these tissues. There are cross-links between collagen fibers, which provide strength and stability. Pro-gesterone causes these cross-links to become more pliable but less stable. So if you have a history of chronic back pain or other joint instability, be aware that you are at an increased risk for injury during pregnancy. Also, this relaxation can allow micromovement to occur and may exacerbate underlying joint dysfunction.

Autoimmune Diseases (Lupus, Rheumatoid Arthritis, Psoriatic Arthritis, Sjögren's Syndrome)

Other conditions that impact the chances of getting pregnant and having a healthy pregnancy are autoimmune diseases that primar-ily affect joints. These include lupus, rheumatoid arthritis, psoriatic arthritis, and Sjögren's syndrome, to name some of the most com-mon. Systemic lupus erythematosus (SLE) can result in a condition called antiphospholipid antibody syndrome (APS), which increases the risk of life-threatening blood clots during pregnancy, as well as the risk of pregnancy complications like miscarriage, stillbirth, and preeclampsia. If you have SLE or APS, blood thinners such as enoxaparin or heparin with aspirin are generally recommended to improve your pregnancy outcomes. When dealing with any auto-immune condition, it is good to have your condition in remission or under the best control possible, preferably with your last flare at least a year in the past. Let your rheumatologist know that you are actively seeking pregnancy. Some medications used for these conditions are not conducive to pregnancy and may need to be stopped for a few months before trying to conceive.

Also, autoimmune diseases travel together. This means that having one autoimmune disease increases the risk of others. If you are in this situation, ensure that your thyroid and ovaries (common targets of autoimmune disease) are in good working order. And if you have evidence of diminished ovarian reserve, time is unfortunately not your friend. In the event you are reading this book because you either need or want IVF and you have an autoimmune disease, consider banking your eggs or embryos to "freeze" your biological clock.

NEUROLOGICAL SYSTEM

The neurological system consists of the brain, spinal cord, and peripheral nerves. If you are considering pregnancy and have any congenital or chronic issues with your neurological system, it is good to let your neurologist know that you are trying to conceive. It is common that women with congenital malformations of the brain, such as hydrocephalus, who are trying to conceive may not have had a recent visit with a neurologist. If so, this is the time to schedule a consult with a neurologist. Hydrocephalus and pseudo-tumor cerebri, a condition characterized by increased pressure inside the skull, can worsen during pregnancy as a result of hormonal changes and changes in fluid balance within the body due to increased blood volume. It is advisable to have a neurologist who is familiar with your specific clinical situation as part of your team during your fertility journey.

Spinal Cord Injury

Spinal cord injuries, unfortunately, affect over 17,000 Americans and between 250,000 to 500,000 people globally each year.[9] If you are a woman with a spinal cord injury pursuing pregnancy, you should visit with a maternal-fetal medicine physician to discuss risks, including blood clots due to immobility and possible need for a cesarean section (C-section). Men who are affected by spinal cord injuries may have issues with ejaculation, though that depends on the severity and level of the injury. If you are seeking IVF and the male sperm source has been affected by a spinal cord injury, a semen analysis is important to see if medical or surgical procedures are necessary to acquire viable sperm for fertilization.

Seizure Disorders

Seizure disorders are another health concern when entering pregnancy, and it is best if your seizures are well controlled before you try to conceive. Having seizures during pregnancy can be quite risky for you as well as for the baby. With well-controlled disease, however, the prognosis is quite good. If you are on anticonvulsants, your fertility specialist needs to know. Some antiseizure medications affect the metabolism of folic acid. Folic acid is necessary to minimize the risk of neural tube defects such as spina bifida and anencephaly. In these situations, you should take 4,000 mcg (4 mg) of folic acid daily instead of the standard recommendation of 400 to 800 mcg (standard prenatal vitamins contain 800 mcg). Because certain anticonvulsants are also not advised during pregnancy, it's best to let your neurologist know you're planning to be pregnant, so that you can get on an appropriate and safe regimen.

Multiple Sclerosis

Multiple sclerosis (MS) is an autoimmune disease of the central nervous system. It tends to develop in women between ages fifteen and fifty, and thus it can have a significant impact on decisions made during the reproductive years. Like many other autoimmune diseases, it may improve during pregnancy as a result of hormonal changes, though this is not guaranteed.[10] Some medications, like interferon-beta and natalizumab, may be used prior to conception and through certain weeks of pregnancy with less risk. Fingolimod and teriflunomide have high risks of birth defects and should be avoided during pregnancy, while others like cladribine, alemtuzumab, and ocrelizumab require washout times prior to conception to be safe.[11] Because the course of MS is not certain during pregnancy, it is important to have an established neurologist work with your REI and obstetrician to ensure the best outcomes for you and your baby.

Hypothalamic Amenorrhea

Certain parts of the human brain are very important for reproduction, specifically the hypothalamus and pituitary gland. The hypothalamus sends signals through the hormone GnRH to the pituitary. The pituitary produces LH and FSH, which signal the ovaries to grow follicles or ovulate. The pituitary also secretes thyroid-stimulating hormone and prolactin, which will be discussed in more detail later in this chapter. Some women seeking IVF may have a condition called hypothalamic amenorrhea (HA), where the hypothalamus does not appropriately produce GnRH; this often results in absent or rare periods. Women with HA usually have very low FSH and LH levels. If HA is suspected, you should have an MRI of the brain (specifically in the areas of the hypothalamus and pituitary) to ensure there is not a structural issue. For improved follicular response, women with GnRH-related amenorrhea are typically prescribed menotropins, which have both FSH and LH activity.

MENTAL HEALTH

Mental health and well-being are *always* very important, especially when trying to conceive and while pregnant. We understand that infertility is a struggle, and it is known that a diagnosis of infertility can be as devastating as a diagnosis of cancer. It is normal to go through the grief process while working on your fertility challenge. Your partner is likely facing the same fears and struggles but may be at a different stage than you are, and that is okay. It is common to need some emotional support during this time. So if you need to see a counselor or seek medical intervention for your mental health, we strongly encourage you to do so.

Many people think they should not be on any medications during fertility treatment or pregnancy. However, the best pregnancy outcomes happen when mental health is good and the psyche is healthy. So while some medications should be avoided, there are quite a few that can be used with little risk.

Good mental health doesn't happen in a vacuum. Ask for help if you need it. We truly want you, your partner, and your future baby to have the best chances possible!

Anxiety and Depression

For people with anxiety or depression, most selective serotonin reuptake inhibitors (SSRIs) are considered safe in pregnancy, especially when both risks and benefits are taken into account, and many have been studied for decades. All SSRIs have risks in pregnancy, including the risk of heart, neural tube, and abdominal wall defects, and the risk of neonatal withdrawal.[12] Because some SSRIs may carry more risk than others, it is best to discuss your medication with your REI specialist and the prescribing physician. Buproprion (Wellbutrin), a common antidepressant and medication used in smoking cessation, is generally not recommended in pregnancy if other options are available and effective. For anxiety, nonmedical treatments may be appropriate. If medication is required, choices can be more limited. Short-acting benzodiazepines (anxiety-relieving medications like alprazolam [Xanax]) are also commonly avoided. These medications increase the risk of miscarriage, low birth weight, and neonatal withdrawal.[13] They can also impair the motor and cognitive development of the growing child in utero.[14] Buspirone (BuSpar), an antianxiety medication that acts by different mechanisms than benzodiazepines, is often used in pregnancy and is considered safe. If you have an anxiety disorder, it can be quite effective at preventing anxiety attacks.

Control of anxiety and depression, whether through counseling, meditation, or prescribed medications, definitively improves pregnancy outcomes. It promotes maternal well-being and quality of life during pregnancy. It also positively impacts prenatal health behaviors and reduces the risk of preterm birth, low birth weight, and postpartum depression.[15] Young children's behavioral, cognitive, and emotional development is improved with good maternal mental health.[16]

Bipolar Disorder

For those who live with bipolar disorder, it is essential that this condition is well controlled before pursuing pregnancy and that your physician is aware of your plans. Hormonal fluctuations during fertility treatment and pregnancy can impact your resilience against potential stressors that can trigger manic or hypomanic episodes. Also, having a good support system, with family, friends, or support groups, is imperative in making your fertility journey safe for you and your baby, as it is often hard to see the early signs of an episode within oneself.

Post-Traumatic Stress Disorder

Post-traumatic stress disorder (PTSD) can significantly impact your fertility care. If you struggle with PTSD, let your REI specialist know what your triggers tend to be. That way, your IVF team can help you through this very personal process in a way that will ease your anxieties and improve your journey.

Eating Disorders

If you have a history of an eating disorder, especially anorexia or bulimia, you must let your REI specialist know. It is important that eating disorders are under good control for you and your baby to get adequate nutrition during pregnancy. Even if you had the active disorder a long time ago, eating disorders can affect the communication signals between the brain and the ovary long after you've recovered. You are more likely to need gonadotropins with LH activity, and you are more likely to be unable to produce an endogenous (within your own body) LH surge. This is especially important in IVF, as you may not be a suitable candidate for a leuprolide trigger. Because you may require an hCG trigger, your physician may need to stimulate your ovaries more gently to reduce the risk of OHSS.

Substance Abuse

Substance abuse is widespread in the population. It is estimated that in the United States, about 20.4 percent of Americans who drink alcohol have an alcohol use disorder, 57.3 million Americans use nicotine products, and 21.4 percent of those over age twelve have used illicit drugs or misused prescription drugs in the last year.[17] We cannot stress enough that substance abuse can have a significant negative impact on fertility, and this applies to both partners. Treat your body as a temple; the things you put in definitely affect what comes out.

GASTROINTESTINAL SYSTEM

The gastrointestinal (GI) system starts at your mouth. It extends down your throat to your stomach, which connects to your small intestine, which in turn connects to your large intestine, which ends with your anus. Abnormalities within your GI tract can have a significant impact on fertility and pregnancy outcomes.

When seeking pregnancy, people are often nervous about routine dental care. Know that healthy teeth and gums are correlated to better pregnancy outcomes and other important health outcomes as you age. So if you are due for a cleaning, go for it! If you are post-transfer and due for X-rays, you can be shielded with a heavy lead drape, or you can choose to pass until your next check-up. If you are having a dental emergency and need antibiotics or a procedure requiring local anesthetic, consult with your OB/GYN. Many pain medications and antibiotics can be used safely during pregnancy.

GERD

Gastroesophageal reflux disease, or GERD, affects men and women of all ages. The good news is this does not have effects on the pregnancy. The bad news is that GERD will likely get worse, not better, in pregnancy. Progesterone, one of the main hormones of pregnancy, is a smooth muscle relaxant. Your entire gastrointestinal system is lined with smooth muscle. When the sphincter between the stomach and esophagus relaxes, this can allow reflux of gastric contents into the esophagus. If you are struggling with GERD before pregnancy, talk to your gastroenterologist about a preventative medication that is safe during pregnancy.

Constipation

The relaxed smooth muscle throughout the GI tract is also the culprit if you are experiencing increased constipation. The best things to do are to increase hydration and fiber. The osmotic laxative polyethylene glycol 3350 (MiraLAX) is safe during pregnancy. And we are huge fans of prunes, whether in the form of the dried fruit or as prune juice over crushed ice (it isn't half bad)! Keep things moving, because constipation will make you unnecessarily miserable.

Autoimmune GI Diseases (Ulcerative Colitis, Crohn's Disease, Celiac Disease)

Autoimmune GI diseases such as ulcerative colitis (UC), Crohn's disease, or celiac disease should be under excellent control before conception. UC and Crohn's are prone to flare-ups during pregnancy, especially during the first trimester. These can be characterized by abdominal pain, diarrhea, rectal bleeding, fatigue, and weight loss. Proper control before pregnancy can help minimize the risk of flares during pregnancy. Malabsorption can also occur with poorly controlled UC or Crohn's, which can lead to nutritional deficiencies for mother and baby. These can impact fetal growth and well-being. The risk of pregnancy complications, including gestational diabetes, preeclampsia, and clotting disorders, increases when UC or Crohn's is not well managed. The risk of C-section is also higher in people with these conditions.[18]

Celiac disease, in particular, should be under good dietary control going into a pregnancy. If you have celiac disease and do not follow a strict gluten-free diet, this can cause damage to the villi within the small intestine. Villi increase the surface area of the intestine, maximizing the absorption of nutrients. If the villi are damaged, it can lead to malabsorption and thus to nutritional deficiencies in the mother and baby. This increases the risk of miscarriage, preterm delivery, low birth weight, stillbirth, and C-section.[19]

ENDOCRINE SYSTEM

The endocrine system is the system of glands throughout your body that produce hormones. Hormones are simply chemical messengers produced by one part of the body to tell another part to do a specific job. The top three endocrine conditions that can affect pregnancy success are thyroid disease, hyperprolactinemia, and diabetes.

Thyroid Disease

The thyroid gland, located in the neck, is the major metabolism gland in the body. It can be underactive (hypothyroidism) or overactive (hyperthyroidism). Either of these can make it more challenging to get pregnant or stay pregnant, and normal thyroid levels are important for fetal neurodevelopment.

When you are having your thyroid checked, the most important hormone is thyroid-stimulating hormone (TSH). TSH is a hormone produced in the pituitary gland that tells the thyroid gland to make thyroid hormones, mainly T3 and T4. TSH is the best marker of thyroid health, especially during pregnancy.

If TSH is elevated, the brain works harder to get the thyroid to do its job. In this case, thyroid supplementation, usually levothyroxine (Synthroid, Tirosint), will be prescribed. It can take time for TSH levels to stabilize when starting or changing thyroid hormone supplementation. Levels are checked every four to eight weeks until the target range is reached, and then adjustments will be made to keep your TSH level at less than 2–2.5 mIU/L. The actual amount of thyroid hormone needed will vary based on how much your thyroid may be producing and your body weight. The more you weigh, the more thyroid hormone supplementation you will likely need.

Sometimes you may have a condition called subclinical hypothyroidism. This happens when the TSH is in a borderline zone (2.5–4.1 mIU/L). If you have thyroid antibodies, specifically thyroid peroxidase (TPO) antibodies, you may be advised to start a low dose of thyroid supplementation to have the best pregnancy outcome.

Hyperthyroidism, a condition in which you have too much thyroid hormone, is much less common than hypothyroidism. Hyperthyroidism can be caused by antibodies, either TPO antibodies or antithyroglobulin antibodies. Hyperthyroidism is commonly called Graves' disease. In Graves' disease, additional symptoms, such as the presence of a goiter (enlarged thyroid) or exophthalmos (bulging eyes), may occur. Hyperthyroidism is often first treated with oral medication such as methimazole or propylthiouracil (PTU). If the oral medications don't work or you have reactions to the medications, you may be advised to have surgery to remove your thyroid or use a substance called radioactive iodine (RAI). RAI is used to chemically damage the thyroid cells and usually results in your becoming hypothyroid. When RAI is used, it is advised not to get pregnant for six months. This allows all the RAI to dissipate from your system and lets you achieve normal thyroid levels with thyroid supplementation.

Thyroid activity can affect the risk of miscarriage. Adequate levels of thyroid hormone are necessary for fetal brain development.

Pituitary Adenoma and Prolactin Disorders

Prolactin is a hormone produced by the pituitary gland. It stimulates the production of breast milk after delivery. However, if it is high at other times, it can make your periods irregular, impede your chances of pregnancy, and increase your risk of miscarriage. Often, during your fertility evaluation, prolactin levels may be checked. Lots of things can make a prolactin level transiently elevated, such as recent intercourse, nipple stimulation, certain medications, and eating before your blood draw. If your screening prolactin level is elevated, you will be advised to repeat the blood draw while fasting (drinking water is okay) with no intercourse, exercise, or nipple stimulation for twenty-four hours before your test. If it remains elevated, you should have MRI imaging done of the pituitary gland. We know this can be a little nerve-racking, but it is important. If there is a growth, it is likely a microprolactinoma — small (less than 10 mm) and inconsequential. A growth larger than 10 mm, a macroprolactinoma, is very unusual. If imaging shows a macroprolactinoma, you may be advised to visit an ophthalmologist to have your visual fields tested. The pituitary sits right where the optic nerves crisscross in the brain. If the growth compresses the optic nerve, you may have some deficits in your peripheral vision, which can be dangerous, especially when driving. In the rare case that you are found to have a macroprolactinoma, you may be advised to see a surgeon to have the growth removed. Believe it or not, this is usually performed through the nose!

Now, back to common things. If your prolactin level is elevated and there is either no growth on the pituitary or a microadenoma, you will be started on medication, either cabergoline or bromocriptine (bromocriptine is an older medication that tends to have more side effects). Once you have a normal prolactin level, you will continue the medication until you get pregnant. When pregnancy is achieved, these medications are discontinued, as it is normal in pregnancy to have elevated prolactin levels. When postpartum and after you wean a breastfed child, you should have your levels rechecked to see if you still need medication.

Diabetes

In the United States, 38.4 million people have diabetes, and 97.6 million people have prediabetes.[20] Diabetes has three different forms. Type 1 diabetes is an autoimmune disease in which the pancreas stops making insulin, which is required for your body to utilize glucose for energy. Type 2 diabetes is when your body does not efficiently use insulin to normalize glucose levels. This is the most common form of diabetes. The third type, gestational diabetes, is a form of diabetes that develops during pregnancy and can cause serious complications for both baby and mother.

Prediabetes is a condition in which blood sugar levels are higher than normal (HgbA1C > 5.6%) but lower than the threshold for a diabetes diagnosis (HgbA1C ≥ 6.5%). Hemoglobin A1C (HgbA1C) is a marker of your average blood sugar over the past three months and is often used to diagnose and monitor diabetes.

With any form of diabetes or prediabetes, you are encouraged to get your blood sugar under excellent control. Especially in the first trimester, high blood sugar is associated with a higher risk of birth defects, particularly heart defects. If you have uncontrolled prediabetes when you conceive, your risk of gestational diabetes is 25.4 times that of someone who has normal blood sugar levels. Also, women who have gestational diabetes are 76.1 times more likely to develop type 2 diabetes.[21] If you have diabetes or gestational diabetes while pregnant, your child is at increased risk of being large for gestational age, which can cause complications at the time of delivery, including your baby having low blood sugar right after delivery (requiring care in the neonatal intensive care unit [NICU]), increased risk of childhood and adult obesity, and increased risk that your child may develop diabetes.[22]

If you need to get better control of your blood sugars, the first step is to modify your diet and increase your exercise. A lower-carb Mediterranean-style diet is a good starting point. We also recommend seeing a nutritionist, who can advise you on altering your dietary habits to succeed. As to exercise, you don't have to join a gym or train for a triathlon; you just need to get moving more. Take a walk, climb the stairs at work, or go for a swim.

If you currently take or need to start medications to control blood sugar, these will need to be prescribed with pregnancy in mind. The gold standard for treating diabetes in pregnancy is insulin because it helps maintain the tightest control of blood sugar with the lowest risk to the baby. Patients on oral medications like metformin (a medication to sensitize cells throughout the body to the actions of insulin) or glipizide may switch over to insulin as soon as they know they are pregnant. Frequently, patients attempting pregnancy will switch to insulin to minimize medication exposures during pregnancy. That said, maintaining blood sugar control differs in each patient, and discussing the best approach for you with your physician(s) is important.

More and more frequently, patients with type 2 diabetes are prescribed a class of medications called GLP-1 agonists, such as Ozempic or Mounjaro. These medications can help patients get excellent blood sugar control. As they are neuroendocrine modulators and we have very little information on how they impact embryological development, if you are taking these medications, you should be transitioned to other methods of diabetic control before going through the IVF process.

———

In conclusion, you need to make sure your health is good before seeking IVF and pregnancy. Chronic medical conditions should be under good control. If you have not seen a physician to manage your condition in a few years, now is the time to make that appointment. If you take medications, talk to your REI specialist and prescribing physicians to see if you are receiving optimal treatment. Don't wait until you are pregnant to get on the regimen you plan to follow during pregnancy. High-risk obstetricians (maternal-fetal medicine docs) specialize in managing complex medical conditions during pregnancy and will be a valuable resource to you during pregnancy and sometimes during preconception counseling. Remember that if you have ovulated or had an embryo transfer, it is best to consider yourself pregnant until proven otherwise. Your body will be home to a growing baby soon enough — make it the best home you can provide!

CHAPTER 5

· · · · · · · · · · · · · · · · ·

Lifestyle Changes That Benefit Mom and Baby

From conception, your baby will share everything you eat, drink, or breathe for the next nine months. Your lifestyle choices before you get pregnant impact your baby. Changing your lifestyle to ensure the best possible chances of a healthy pregnancy is a group effort between you, your doctor, and your fertility team. It may be challenging to change some of your habits, but there is no better reason than a baby to make those changes.

This chapter will primarily discuss the big challenges that face many of us — smoking, marijuana use, excess weight, and alcohol use. Many women are motivated to change bad habits when pregnant, which is certainly something to applaud. Since you will be doing IVF soon, consider making lifestyle changes that will improve your health *before* you start treatment. Remember, your actions impact you *and* your future baby. Having optimal health before pregnancy is essential.

CIGARETTES AND VAPING

If you are currently smoking cigarettes or e-cigarettes, *stop*. Information about the negative impact of smoking during pregnancy has been around for many years. Vaping, on the other hand, is newer and has sometimes been perceived as a "healthier" way of using nicotine, but that is not the case. In addition, marijuana is now legal in many areas of the country, and its use has increased dramatically. Beware — don't mistake the legal use of marijuana for safe use in pregnancy.

When you use nicotine, your embryo, fetus, and baby use nicotine with you — not a nice picture for the baby album. It doesn't matter if the nicotine is from cigarettes, vaping, patches, or gum — nicotine is nicotine. If you plan to do IVF, the other reason to stop nicotine is to improve your chances of achieving a successful pregnancy. *Nicotine use (including exposure to secondhand smoke) will decrease your odds of having a successful pregnancy by 40 to 50 percent.* That means if you are young and have a good egg count, your chance of having a baby in your arms will decrease from 60 percent to 30 percent. That's huge!

Smoking harms your overall fertility. We have known for years that patients who smoke have a lower egg number and go through menopause at an earlier age. Smokers have a higher chance of infertility, a higher risk of miscarriage, and a higher chance of having a baby die in the first year of life. While this information sounds like gloom and doom, remember that regardless of your past, your actions today have the power to change the outcome and optimize IVF success.

If a better chance of a successful IVF outcome hasn't convinced you to change your bad habits, here are some other reasons to throw your cigarettes in the trash. Preterm birth is two times higher in smokers compared to the general population. Maybe delivering early sounds good, but your baby needs nine months to develop fully. If you stop smoking, you can significantly increase the likelihood of that happening. Quitting smoking is one of the few ways to reduce the possibility of having a baby too early. If you smoke, you have a 400 percent increase in your risk of premature rupture of membranes (breaking your water), which leads to delivering early.[1]

Other conditions associated with cigarette smoking include having a low-birth-weight baby, stillbirth, and having a baby with malformations. About one in five babies weighing less than six pounds are born to women who smoke, and there is a 50 percent greater risk of having a stillborn baby if you smoke.[2] Evidence also suggests that nicotine is teratogenic, which means it can cause malformations in the baby. Specifically, it can increase facial malformations, including cleft lip, a condition where the upper lip fuses incorrectly during fetal development. In addition, it can cause a division inside the mouth (cleft palate), which makes it difficult for the baby to suck or eat when it is born and which requires surgery.

As we noted earlier, the alternative to smoking cigarettes, vaping, hasn't lived up to its initial promise as a "healthier" habit. Vaping, like the use of cigarettes, has been shown to increase preterm birth rates and increase the risk of low-birth-weight babies. Not very much is known about the other impacts of vaping. It would be unethical to determine the effects of vaping on pregnancy by designing a large study where half of the pregnant women vape and half don't. Instead, we assess the impact of vaping on pregnancies by evaluating babies from mothers who continue to do it. And that takes time.

In studies evaluating cigarette smoking, nicotine appears to be the culprit causing problems. The amount of nicotine absorbed through e-cigarette use is about the same as in traditional cigarette use — although some studies suggest that women who vape may be more likely to have higher nicotine levels, depending on how much they puff. If used correctly, nicotine patches probably result in lower nicotine levels than cigarettes or vaping.[3] To be clear, they are *all* terrible for your baby. Nicotine causes constriction of blood vessels in the placenta, reducing blood flow to your unborn child. It also increases the carbon monoxide in your bloodstream, depriving your baby of adequate oxygen. The nicotine in vapes likely has the same harmful effects on pregnancies.

MARIJUANA

Marijuana is legal in many states and is accepted by many as a recreational drug. Marijuana use exposes you to a couple of compounds you have probably heard about. Tetrahydrocannabinol (THC) gives you the psychotropic effect. Cannabidiol (CBD), a phytocannabinoid, is another breakdown product but does not have the same psychotropic effect. CBD is also sold separately, usually containing a very low amount of THC or none; often it is diluted with oil from hemp or coconuts. CBD can affect neurons and cognition. Unfortunately, the mechanism of action for CBD is not fully known, and so we do not know what its impact is on pregnancy.[4]

We all have cannabinoid receptors, which bind a chemical produced by our bodies called anandamide. These receptors send signals to the brain to regulate several bodily functions, including sleep, appetite, movement — and pregnancy.[5] The body's cannabinoid receptors play essential roles in uterine receptivity, implantation, and embryo development.[6] Even cravings for dark chocolate may be related to anandamide. Once you start to eat that candy bar, anandamide is released, causing you to feel a sense of calm (Godiva, here I come!).

Unfortunately, THC from marijuana does not have the same chill effect on your baby as it does on you. THC from marijuana can harm placental growth. It also makes it difficult for your baby to absorb folic acid. There is even concern that THC can enter your breast milk and pass to your baby.[7] Most of this research studied women who smoked marijuana; unfortunately, we do not have similar studies on the edible forms that have become more available, but because these expose you to THC and CBD also, we recommend that you not use them either.

Furthermore, women who use marijuana may also smoke and drink, contributing negatively to pregnancy outcomes.

HEALTHY WEIGHT FOR
MAMA = HEALTHY BABY

Weight loss is not an easy topic to discuss, but if your doctor can't be honest with you, who can? Whether you are overweight or underweight, there can be adverse side effects if you are not at a healthy weight. Being overweight in particular can cause significant problems in pregnancy, including miscarriage, gestational diabetes, high blood pressure, labor complications, and even death of the mother.[8] The heavier the mother, the more challenging pregnancy complications can be.

What Is a Healthy Weight?

So, what is the optimal weight? It depends. The best way we currently have to evaluate weight is body mass index (BMI), which takes both height and weight into consideration. Some argue that BMI is not an ideal way to assess all people. For example, larger people may have larger bone mass, and smaller people may have smaller bone mass. In addition, muscular people (such as athletes or those who work out frequently) are often heavier because muscle cells weigh more than fat cells. While it's true that evaluating weight with BMI is not perfect, it is still the best way to compare individuals with different heights and weights.

An optimal muscle-to-fat ratio must be present for a woman to produce an egg each month, but that optimal ratio varies among individuals. Having an adequate fat supply was necessary when the earliest humans fought for survival—your body did not want to release an egg and get you pregnant if you needed your energy for survival. That same rudimentary system is still in operation today, despite all the changes in humans' lives, and can impact ovulation.

For the healthiest possible pregnancy, the goal is to strive for a normal BMI. Women with a BMI between 18.5 and 24.9 kg/m^2 have the lowest risk of pregnancy complications.[9] If your BMI is less than 18.5 kg/m^2 (underweight) when you become pregnant, your doctor will probably want you to gain more weight during pregnancy, as women who are underweight are at higher risk of preterm birth and having babies with low birth weight.[10] If you are overweight, meaning a BMI of 25 to 29.9 kg/m^2, you will be asked to gain less weight during your pregnancy, and even less if your BMI is over 30 kg/m^2. Ideally, it is best to work on your BMI before pregnancy. In particular, women who are overweight should not shed pounds during pregnancy but rather maintain a constant weight. If a woman has a significant amount of weight loss during pregnancy, the breakdown products of fat cells can interfere with fetal brain development. That is why we do not want women who have recently had weight loss surgery to get pregnant. If you have that type of surgery, you should not get pregnant for at least one year after surgery, and your weight loss should be stabilized.

Losing Weight

It is okay to get help if you are having trouble losing weight. There are nutritionists whom you can see in person. Some drop-in clinics even employ nutritionists to help with weight loss. Online weight loss companies can also make nutritionists available to you through telemedicine visits. One of the easiest ways to start losing weight is by eliminating the one thing you know is sabotaging your diet. For some people, it may be candy; for others, it may be pasta or bread. Anything that increases carbohydrates in your diet will make it harder to lose weight.

If you are losing weight under the direction of a physician, in addition to a healthy diet and exercise, you may choose to use certain medications or procedures to help. Metformin, a member of a class of medications called biguanides, has historically been used to help control blood sugar in those with prediabetes or diabetes by improving the body's response to insulin. Metformin can aid in weight loss by decreasing appetite, improving insulin sensitivity, decreasing fat absorption in the intestines, and changing the metabolic processes that determine how carbs and fats are used for energy.[11] Metformin is safe for women to continue during pregnancy and may reduce the risk of gestational diabetes.[12] Note, however, that metformin is usually not advisable for men trying to conceive due to possible risks of birth defects, most commonly in the cardiac, genitourinary, musculoskeletal, and gastrointestinal systems.[13]

Phentermine is an appetite suppressant commonly used as a short-term medical adjunct for weight loss. It stimulates the secretion of certain neurotransmitters in the brain, such as norepinephrine, to suppress appetite. It should not be used in pregnancy and should be discontinued before trying to conceive. Phentermine clears the body quickly and should be out of your system about four days after the last dose.[14]

Two newer classes of medications have hit the weight loss industry in the past few years, GLP-1 receptor agonists (semaglutide [Ozempic, Wegovy, Rybelsus]) and dual GLP-1/GIP receptor agonists (tirzepatide [Zepbound, Mounjaro]). These medications help weight loss by improving blood glucose levels and stimulating satiety (a feeling of fullness). They are some of the most effective medications for achieving weight loss.[15] However, unlike phentermine, they linger for quite some time in the body and must be discontinued two months before conception.

Increasing physical activity aids in weight loss and helps you have a healthier pregnancy.[16] It is best to start working out before you get pregnant. But don't get too caught up worrying about exactly how long you exercise in each session. Anything that causes you to exert additional energy will be beneficial. Focus on getting healthy instead of losing weight. Even if you do not have time to go to the gym, think of ways to increase your number of steps daily. If the weather is nice, walk around the block with your partner as you catch up on each other's day. Maintain a quick pace; you're aiming to be slightly breathless while sharing that funny story from work. Make exercise a priority. It takes about six weeks for an activity to become a habit. If you are successful, you will be glad you've done it. Another benefit: women who are fit going into pregnancy have a shorter labor.[17]

Weight loss surgeries such as gastric bypass and gastric sleeve are also popular among adults in their reproductive years who need additional help losing significant weight. The results can be quite dramatic, and these surgeries should strongly be considered if your BMI is greater than 40 kg/m^2. If you have had weight loss surgery, you are more likely to have short-term vitamin and mineral deficiencies, which puts a new pregnancy at increased risk of growth and development problems. Talk to your gastric surgeon about the best type of vitamin supplements that will enable you to maintain high levels of folic acid and other necessary micronutrients. You should start taking these supplements at least three months before trying to conceive.

Diabetes

If you have diabetes or prediabetes, ensuring it is under optimal control before you conceive is essential. High glucose levels increase the risk that your baby may have birth defects. Furthermore, babies of women with poorly controlled diabetes often have low glucose levels at birth. They will likely need to stay in the neonatal intensive care unit after delivery so that their glucose and insulin levels can be monitored and regulated.

> Making simple changes in your diet can significantly impact prediabetes. Try to snack throughout the day rather than eating large meals. Snacks high in fiber or protein tend to keep your insulin levels constant. Preventing big swings in insulin minimizes cravings that can sabotage your diet.

Gestational diabetes, as we noted in Chapter 4, is a condition women get only during pregnancy. When the mother has gestational diabetes, babies can gain too much weight. Weight gain in babies is primarily seen in the neck and shoulders, making it more likely for them to have shoulder dystocia — when the baby is too big to come out of the birth canal. Often, shoulder dystocia is not recognized until delivery, when the baby is already in the birth canal; this puts the baby in danger and often leads to an emergency C-section. Some women with gestational diabetes will have an elective C-section to minimize the risk of the baby getting stuck in the birth canal due to their large neck and chest. Babies of women with poorly controlled gestational diabetes are also likely to have low blood glucose levels at birth, just like babies of women with poorly controlled type 1 or type 2 diabetes. Women with gestational diabetes will no longer have diabetes once they have delivered, but they do have a higher risk of developing diabetes in the future.

High Blood Pressure

High blood pressure can also develop during pregnancy, and it's more likely to happen if you're overweight. You probably know many people who have high blood pressure and do not seem to have any side effects at present. However, in this situation, you and your baby will be impacted by this condition. It can also turn into a more severe condition known as preeclampsia. Preeclampsia occurs only in pregnancy and affects both mom and baby. In extreme cases, it can lead to maternal kidney damage, worsening high blood pressure, and even seizures. If severe preeclampsia occurs, the baby has to be delivered regardless of gestational age. Preeclampsia tends to occur in a woman's first pregnancy, and it is more likely in women who are at the extremes of reproductive age (very young or much older) and women who are obese. Fortunately, most women who develop preeclampsia with their first pregnancy do not develop it in subsequent pregnancies.

Even if you don't develop preeclampsia, high blood pressure during pregnancy impacts the baby by decreasing blood flow to the placenta. Your blood is the source of nutrition for the baby, and your blood vessels are the pipes that take blood to the placenta. When you have high blood pressure, those blood vessels constrict, and the placenta doesn't receive as much of the nutrient-filled blood as your baby needs. If this happens early in pregnancy, it can impact the growth and development of the placenta. If placental growth is affected early in pregnancy, your baby may not grow well and have a higher risk of other complications, including stillbirth. It's a scary topic, but if you know the risks, you will understand why controlling your blood pressure before and during pregnancy is vital.

Labor Complications

Obesity also increases the risk of labor complications. Complications include a longer labor than usual and infection. When women are obese, fatty tissue in the birth canal can get in the way of the baby's head, making it difficult for the baby to emerge. Once your water breaks, your baby comes into contact with germs from the outside world. Long exposure to this environment before delivery increases the chances of an infection for you and the baby. When that occurs, your doctor may recommend a C-section.

Many women end up with a C-section. However, in the absence of a medical indication for C-section, it is best to deliver the baby the old-fashioned way, through the vagina. Though many C-sections are safe and uneventful, complications can happen, and they are more likely to occur if you are overweight. Doing a C-section on an obese woman is technically more difficult. There are thicker layers of tissue to go through, and lifting the baby out of the pelvis may be challenging for the physician. About 50 percent of your blood supply goes to your uterus when pregnant, and so the longer a C-section takes, the more likely it is you will have continued blood loss, even to the point of needing a blood transfusion. The wound from surgery is less likely to heal well and will have a higher risk of infection. A C-section is a major surgery with a large incision, which can make recovery while caring for a newborn baby challenging; if there are complications, this new phase of life may be even more difficult.

Even though the United States has quality medical care, we still have one of the highest maternal death rates of any developed country. Fortunately, the death of a laboring mom is a rare event, but being overweight can increase that chance. We want you to be around to raise your beautiful new boy or girl!

DON'T MAKE THE BABY W(H)INE!

Many of us don't mind coming home and having a glass of wine. There is usually nothing wrong with that unless you are pregnant or trying to get pregnant. Your baby needs nine months in a pleasant and inviting space. Alcohol is not part of that equation. Is there a safe amount of alcohol? Probably not. Alcohol is not processed in the liver at the same rate for all people. That six-ounce glass of wine may absorb more slowly into your five-foot frame, causing you to feel a little tipsy and slur your speech, while the same amount of wine may not faze your six-foot best friend. The total amount that you drink and the rate at which you drink matter too. Drinking four beers on Saturday—binge drinking—is probably worse than drinking one beer a day for four days because it leads to a high amount of alcohol in your system. Heavy drinking—which is defined as eight or more drinks a week—poses a similar risk to your baby as weekend binge drinking. Another challenge in determining a "safe" level of alcohol is keeping track of what and how much you've consumed.[18] When you go to a bar with your buddies, we doubt you keep track of the details (except maybe vowing never to do a tequila shot again). It's probably best to be the designated driver and refrain from alcohol for the foreseeable future.

What does alcohol do? It circulates quickly to the placenta and then to the baby. Higher concentrations are more likely to cause damage to your developing baby. Alcohol consumption may also cause preterm delivery and delivery of growth-restricted babies. Babies exposed frequently to alcohol can develop fetal alcohol syndrome (FAS). Babies with FAS may have different types of characteristics, so diagnosing them can be challenging. Symptoms seen include abnormalities with facial development, problems with growth, neurological abnormalities, and seizures.[19] Children with FAS tend to have hyperactivity, learning difficulties, and lower intelligence. There is no treatment for this condition other than prevention.

Alcohol doesn't affect your baby just while they're developing in the womb; it also can harm your child at conception and during breastfeeding. Alcohol has been shown to harm cell division and may impact the number of chromosomes in your egg. Because of this, it is a good idea to give up alcohol even when trying to get pregnant. And alcohol you consume can pass through your breast milk to the baby.

With knowledge, there is power, so make a toast to parenthood with your nonalcoholic beverage of choice!

DIAMONDS ARE FOREVER, BUT VACCINES ARE NOT

Just because you had a vaccine as a child does not mean you will have lifelong protection. Pregnant women can get very sick from illnesses that generally have no impact on their nonpregnant counterparts. You may have noticed that medical authorities talk about three "high-risk" groups during flu season: the very young, the elderly, and pregnant women. Most young, healthy women are not used to being included in the high-risk category. However, pregnancy changes everything, including your immune system. Suppression of your immune system is how nature allows you to grow another human within your body. But that same suppression makes it harder to fight germs in your environment.

A good example is chickenpox (varicella). Most of us think of chickenpox as a benign childhood illness. Because of immunosuppression during pregnancy, you are more likely to get infections like chickenpox. Unfortunately, pregnant patients with chickenpox can get ill very quickly with pneumonia; they may end up on a ventilator in the ICU, develop encephalitis (brain inflammation), and even die. Unborn babies exposed to chickenpox can also suffer severe consequences, including facial scarring and brain and limb abnormalities. Fortunately, that does not happen often, but it is clear that vaccines are critical to improve your odds of a healthy pregnancy.

Make sure your vaccinations are up to date before pregnancy. The ones we recommend every year are influenza and, now, the COVID-19 vaccine or booster. There are other vaccines that are often given in childhood, and sometimes by adulthood the immunity they provide has waned; your physician can test to see if you still have adequate immunity to those diseases. Getting a tetanus-diphtheria-pertussis (Tdap) vaccine as a booster is vital if your immunity has waned.[20] You can get Tdap during pregnancy, but getting it before conception is best. It's important to check before you become pregnant whether you are immune to chickenpox; some of us had the disease as a kid, and others were vaccinated. If you are not immune, you will need two doses of the vaccine, one month apart, and you should not get pregnant for one month after the last injection. Another vaccine that may require a booster is measles, mumps, and rubella (MMR).[21] After getting the vaccine, you must wait one month before you can conceive. Like chickenpox, measles, mumps, and rubella can cause severe fetal malformations if you get infected in the first twelve weeks of pregnancy. In addition, a hepatitis B booster or vaccination is recommended before pregnancy for all who are not immune, to prevent complications in newborns and the potential for chronic hepatitis; you will want to have your immunity checked for this too.

YOUR PARTNER'S LIFESTYLE CHOICES MATTER TOO

Male infertility is also negatively impacted by lifestyle choices. Obesity, physical inactivity, alcohol, and the use of marijuana decrease the chance of successful conception.

A retrospective study in men showed a negative correlation between body mass and ejaculate volume, sperm concentration, and morphology.[22] In animal models, diets high in fat affect the structure of sperm and can negatively impact the health of the developing fetus.[23] Sedentary men have been shown to have fewer moving sperm and more malformed sperm.[24] As noted earlier, though, metformin use is discouraged in men whose partners are trying to conceive because of the risk of birth defects.

The effect of alcohol on male reproduction has been more extensively studied than the effect of other substances. An early study showed that over half of men who were heavy drinkers had smaller testes and had partial or complete arrest of sperm production as compared to controls at the time of autopsy.[25] There is also an abnormal increase in estrogen and a decrease in testosterone in men who are alcoholics. In addition, there is a significant decrease in sperm parameters, including count, volume, and motility of normally shaped sperm.[26] The impact of moderate alcohol intake in men is not clear. It has been shown that alcohol intake within the previous five days tends to result in abnormal semen characteristics, which tend to worsen with increased intake.[27] One study evaluated men who drank occasionally versus daily drinkers and further subdivided them into fertile versus infertile men. Fertile men were defined as men who had fathered a pregnancy in the past year. As you might guess, daily drinkers who were infertile had poorer semen quality as compared to the other groups.

Exposure to tobacco may also contribute to infertility in men. Tobacco smoke has been shown to contain over four thousand chemicals, including heavy metals such as lead, cadmium, arsenic, and others that are linked with fetal malformation.[28] These chemicals are routinely inhaled in cigarette smoke and lead to sperm damage from changes at the molecular level.[29] Specifically, there are changes in the structure of the neck and tail of the sperm in heavy smokers.[30] There is also a change in the function of sperm, which is likely to interfere with the sperm's ability to penetrate the egg.[31] Your partner's smoking may have an impact on your fertility too. One study showed that infertility risk increases by as much as 64 percent with exposure to secondhand tobacco smoke.[32]

Smoking marijuana has been shown to have a negative impact on the male reproductive system. Interestingly, cannabinoid receptors are present in Sertoli cells (which produce sperm) and Leydig cells (which produce testosterone), suggesting that cannabis has a direct impact on testosterone and sperm production in the testes.[33] Further proof of the hormonal impact of marijuana was shown when men who chronically smoked marijuana were found to have significantly lower levels of testosterone as compared to controls. When use was stopped, testosterone levels increased.[34] However, other studies have contradicted the results. In a case study with 1,700 participants, it was shown that the use of marijuana is a controllable risk factor for poor sperm morphology.[35] This evidence suggests that your partner's lifestyle choices can significantly impact his health and fertility outcome.

We have covered information in this chapter to get you into tip-top shape for pregnancy. After these changes, what baby would not want to live in your luxurious uterus for nine months? The other lifestyle changes discussed will also make you healthier and more likely to get pregnant with IVF. In the next chapter, you will get the lowdown on supplements that may add an extra punch. Find out which ones give you the most bang for your buck.

CHAPTER 6

. . . .

Supplements That Provide
the Extra Vroom

Stocking up your medicine cabinet can give your eggs and sperm an extra spark, a little vroom. Let's talk about supplements — vitamins, minerals, and antioxidants — you may be wondering about.

Vitamins come from plants and animals; your body just doesn't have the blueprint to make most of them. If you follow a limited diet, you may miss out on some recommended vitamins. Some vitamins are fat-soluble, meaning they are stored in your fat cells; specifically, they are vitamins A, D, E, and K. Most other vitamins are water-soluble, and the excess amount not needed by your body is released in urine. Minerals come from the soil and water. Calcium, iron, and iodine are in this category, among others. Antioxidants (examples include coenzyme Q10 [CoQ10], vitamin C, and vitamin E — yep, some vitamins can also be antioxidants) help defend against harmful substances that weaken the integrity of your cells.

Before you dash to the store or order online, here are a few things you need to know about supplements. Most important to know is that because the FDA doesn't regulate supplements, many supplement manufacturers make false claims about what's actually in those bottles. Fortunately, two independent groups, United States Pharmacopeia (USP) and NSF International, do evaluate and endorse companies that adhere to good manufacturing practices. The supplements you buy should have a USP or NSF verification. That verification means the supplements do not contain harmful ingredients and that the tablets or capsules will dissolve in the body, which is critical for a vitamin to be effective. USP and NSF also require companies seeking verification to comply with stringent manufacturing, packaging, and labeling requirements so that each pill has consistent strength, quality, and purity.

Many companies have turned to manufacturing gummy vitamins to make vitamins more appealing. As yummy as they may be, many gummy vitamins contain more fillers — like gelatin, sucrose, water, and corn syrup — than actual vitamins; that's not harmful to you, but it's not helpful. Also, some important components are difficult to include in a gummy form. Make sure you are getting good-quality supplements with USP or NSF verification to keep you and your future baby healthy.

Now that we have discussed how to find a quality supplement, let's dive into the crucial ones for pregnant or soon-to-be-pregnant women like you.

PRENATAL VITAMINS

Why are prenatal vitamins so important? Prenatals keep soon-to-be-pregnant and pregnant women healthy. They contain vitamins and minerals in quantities specific for pregnant women to increase the chances of having a healthy baby. Thirteen vitamins are essential — A, C, D, E, K, and eight B vitamins. Minerals also sparkle with importance, with iron, calcium, and iodine at the top of the list. Here is a quick rundown of what those vitamins and minerals do for you and your baby.

The B vitamins, often found in nuts, seeds, veggies, and meat, are similar in that most work in some way to break down sugar, fats, carbohydrates, and protein to produce energy. Many B vitamins are also crucial for cell growth and production of blood cells. The B vitamins are nature's overachievers — they're all up in everyone's business, from brainpower to energy. Each B vitamin has another name. In case this comes up at your next trivia night, the names of the B vitamins are B_1 (thiamine), B_2 (riboflavin), B_3 (niacin), B_5 (pantothenic acid), B_6 (pyridoxine), B_7 (biotin), B_9 (folate), and B_{12} (cyanocobalamin).[1]

B_9 (folate) is a favorite of fertility docs everywhere. That is because folic acid is crucial in decreasing the risk of birth defects in the development of the baby's brain and spinal cord, commonly known as neural tube defects. These defects can range from spina bifida, where all or part of the spinal cord is exposed, to anencephaly, where parts of the brain, skull, and scalp do not form. It also can prevent congenital heart defects and cleft lip and palate. It is best to have optimal levels *before* conception, as the critical developmental period is during the first trimester.

The terms "folate," "folic acid," and "5-methyltetrahydrofolate (5-Me-THF)" can often lead to confusion. Let's clarify! "Folate" is best used for the nutrient as it's obtained from sources in your diet, such as dark green leafy vegetables, whole grains, beans, and fresh fruits. Folic acid, found in supplements, is a synthetic form of folate that is more stable and easily absorbed. This is because it comes as a simpler form called a monoglutamate. Dietary folate must be broken down into monoglutamates to enter cells, where the monoglutamates then form a more complex active molecule. It's like disassembling a piece of furniture to get it through the front door and then reassembling it inside the house so you can use it. These assembled molecules, called polyglutamates, undergo chemical changes that convert the molecule to an active form called 5-Me-THF through the enzyme 5,10-methylenetetrahydrofolate reductase (MTHFR).[2]

Many people have heard about concerns regarding variations in the gene that controls production of MTHFR. These variations, called polymorphisms, are very common and may occur in a quarter of the general population.[3] Certain (not all) variations in this gene can affect levels of folate in the blood and increase pregnancy complication risks in the second and third trimesters. So, how should you get an adequate intake of folate to help improve the chances of a healthy pregnancy?

Dietary folate is often insufficient to adequately support the human body for pregnancy, so supplementation with 400–800 mcg of folic acid is recommended. However, balance is key. For those with a personal or family history of neural tube defects, higher dosages are recommended. If you have concerns about adequate MTHFR activity, there is evidence that higher doses of folic acid can overcome decreased activity. But guidelines recommend no more than 1 mg of folic acid daily from supplements or fortified foods. Alternatively, you can take 5-Me-THF, which does not require MTHFR activity.[4] But taking more folic acid is not necessarily better — there are emerging concerns that excessively high folate intake may increase the risk of autism spectrum and other neurocognitive disorders.[5]

Vitamins A, D, and E are also antioxidants. They help tame free radicals — molecules with unpaired electrons searching for a mate — which wreak havoc on your cells.[6] When a free radical attacks one of your cells, that's called oxidative stress. It's like leaving a puppy alone in your house all day. When you get home, the house is a disaster. Free radicals do the same thing to your cells. Antioxidants provide that missing electron and make it less likely that free radicals will harm your cells.

While vitamin A is valuable and has many uses in the body, this vitamin is fat-soluble and can be hard to eliminate from the body if you take too much. Large amounts of vitamin A can result in abnormalities in your baby's development.[7] Like Goldilocks, you don't want too much or too little, just the right amount. Of note, a specific form of vitamin A, retinoic acid, used to treat cystic acne, should never be used when trying to get pregnant, since it has been shown to result in fetal malformations.

Vitamin D is one of the few vitamins our bodies can make when our skin is exposed to sunlight. It takes about twenty minutes of whole-body direct sunlight to get your daily dose (but that can vary depending on your skin tone, the season of the year, and the latitude at which you live). Many people don't have enough sun exposure daily for their bodies to produce the recommended amount. Over a billion people worldwide are vitamin D deficient.[8] Those with obesity and polycystic ovary syndrome (PCOS) are at even higher risk of being vitamin D deficient. Anything that protects your skin from sun exposure, such as sunscreen or melanin in dark skin, prevents you from getting the necessary vitamin D. But don't let your need for sufficient vitamin D trick you into skipping sunscreen. There are safer ways to stay glowing and healthy, like foods fortified with vitamin D or a good supplement. Protect your skin *and* your health — it's a win-win!

Vitamin D plays a key role in reducing insulin resistance, controlling inflammation, and reducing oxidative stress. In the short term, vitamin D deficiency can increase the risk of type 2 diabetes and gestational diabetes. In the long term, it can increase cholesterol levels and the risk of heart disease.[9] In regard to pregnancy outcomes, vitamin D supplementation likely reduces the risk of preeclampsia and gestational diabetes as well as the risk of having a baby with low birth weight.[10]

Vitamin E helps support your immune system and increases blood flow to your uterus, making your endometrium lush and welcoming for an embryo transfer. Some doctors even use it to help grow the endometrium. As with vitamin A, we don't recommend taking extra doses of vitamin E, since it can be stored in fat cells, and too much can be problematic.

Vitamin C, like vitamin E, may boost your immune system, and it also helps you absorb the iron in your prenatal vitamin. Vitamin C may decrease the risk of certain types of cancer and help make your brain less foggy — bye-bye, baby brain!

The word "mineral" may make you think more about your eighth-grade earth science class than having a baby, but many minerals do essential work in your body. Iron, for example, is vital in carrying oxygen to your developing baby via red blood cells. When you are pregnant, your blood volume increases by 50 percent, as noted earlier, and increased iron intake helps red blood cells multiply. Heme iron, the kind of iron found in meat, is absorbed better than non-heme iron, which comes from plant foods — think beans, lentils, and chickpeas.[11] Many prenatal vitamins contain iron because it is an important mineral during pregnancy. Unfortunately, it has a side effect you should know about — constipation. If you are prone to constipation or find that you are not as regular as you once were, think about taking a stool softener or adding extra fiber to your diet to compensate for that unpleasant side effect.

Minerals like calcium and iodine, along with vitamins D and K, help bone formation. Your baby will start to make solid bones around twelve weeks. If you don't add calcium to your diet or supplement, your baby will steal some of the calcium from your own bones and teeth. (Dentists fill lots of cavities in pregnant women for that reason.)

DHA (docosahexaenoic acid) is a type of healthy fat that plays a key role in every cell in the body, and it's especially important during pregnancy. Found in large amounts in the brain and eyes, DHA supports fetal development and may help reduce the risk of early delivery.

Studies show that when a fetus has more DHA, it can lead to better vision in the first year of life.[12] In the third trimester, the baby's body starts absorbing large amounts of DHA, which might also influence the beginning of labor.[13] Taking DHA supplements during pregnancy has been linked to longer pregnancies and a lower chance of preterm birth, possibly because of its anti-inflammatory effects.[14] In 2010, the US Department of Health and Human Services suggested that people eat eight to twelve ounces of seafood each week to get enough DHA, but many fall short.[15] That's why the World Association of Perinatal Medicine recommends that pregnant people aim for a daily dose of 200 mg of DHA.[16]

CoQ10

Coenzyme Q10 is an antioxidant with a weird but catchy name that may have a unique role in reproduction and has gotten much attention. It may help with cell division in your most crucial reproductive cell — your egg. Let's talk about what we know, and you can be the judge.

To understand the possible benefits of CoQ10, we must go back to when you were a cuddly newborn in your mother's arms. Back then, you had millions of fresh egg cells, which were brand-new. Since having a baby was not the top priority for your survival, those cells went into hibernation mode to conserve energy, much like your laptop. Over the next decades, some of your cells took a few hits from free radicals. Now, here you are with thirtysomething-year-old egg cells that are not quite as energetic as they used to be. It's time for them to wake up and help you make a baby. But they need lots of energy to do that.

Why do they need so much power? If a cell is going to divide correctly, everything in the cell must divide into two equal parts, including your chromosomes. Twenty-three chromosomes must go in one direction, and twenty-three must go in the other direction during cell division — more to come on that in Chapter 11. That process needs energy. The energy for any cell in your body is from mitochondria, structures in the cell.[17] (Mitochondria are inherited through your maternal cell line. Your mom inherited her mitochondria from her mother, and so on. Who knew that Grandma's mitochondria were more valuable than her china?)

Like a battery producing voltage, mitochondria produce ATP, which provides energy for each cell.[18] Early in your life, before your egg cells go into hibernation, those egg cells make lots of mitochondria to help power them later in life. However, like cell phone batteries, they can lose their charge if they sit around too long. When it is time for the egg to divide, hairlike structures called spindles must form and pull the chromosomes apart.[19] The only fuel for that process and the growing embryo in the first five days of development is from your thirtysomething-year-old mitochondria. Generally, older cells have lower-quality mitochondria with less ATP.[20] When cells have insufficient energy, eggs are less likely to divide correctly and more likely to have an abnormal chromosome number as they age.

Coenzyme Q10 may provide the needed additional power for your egg cells. In an animal study, mitochondrial function and number improved when they received CoQ10 supplements.[21] Another animal study showed that adding mitochondria to a culture with poor-quality eggs increased the number of good-quality embryos compared to ones that did not get the same treatment.[22]

A few studies have been performed with CoQ10 in humans. In one, infertile women received either treatment with 600 mg of

CoQ10 daily for two months or a placebo. After IVF, those who used CoQ10 were more likely to have genetically normal eggs than the other group.[23] However, the study was small, and so it's hard to prove that this finding did not occur due to chance alone. A more recent study evaluated immature eggs in the IVF lab and the impact of CoQ10. Immature eggs have not yet undergone meiosis (recall that this is the process of reducing the number of chromosomes by half so that the egg can be ready to receive a new set of chromosomes from the sperm). The study aimed to see if CoQ10, when added to the culture fluid, would add enough power to do that. The results suggested that adding CoQ10 to the cells in culture helped them divide correctly.[24] A third study evaluated women under age thirty-five with poor ovarian reserve. The women who received CoQ10 for sixty days before egg retrieval had better outcomes in terms of improved egg and embryo quality than women who did not receive CoQ10. Birth rates tended to be higher in the CoQ10 group as well, but that result could have been due to chance.[25] It makes scientific sense that CoQ10 helps produce healthy eggs, and hopefully there will soon be larger and more rigorous studies to guide treatment dose and timing. CoQ10 is certainly one of our favorite supplements. It's like a personal trainer for your eggs and embryos — boosting energy, fighting off stress, and helping them shine their brightest for the big moment!

> A **placebo** is a non-active medication for comparison purposes — essentially a sugar pill.

AND YOU THOUGHT MELATONIN
WAS JUST FOR SLEEP

In recent years, melatonin, a hormone mainly known for its role in sleep, has hit the fertility landscape. Derived from tryptophan (the hormone that makes you sleepy after a big Thanksgiving meal) and serotonin (a hormone that regulates mood, among other things), melatonin is produced in the pineal gland of the brain as well as in eggs and mitochondria.[26] Younger people have higher melatonin levels, but as with many hormones, melatonin levels decline with age.

Melatonin is also a potent antioxidant.[27] Melatonin even stimulates the creation of other antioxidants, such as glutathione. Increasing melatonin intake significantly elevates melatonin levels in the follicular fluid surrounding each egg, surpassing the melatonin level in the blood.[28] It protects ovarian tissue from age-related free radical damage.[29] Ovaries that lack melatonin have increased mitochondrial dysfunction, extensive DNA damage, failure of egg maturation, and depletion of eggs.[30] One study even showed that increased melatonin levels were correlated with normal AMH and FSH levels, further highlighting the potential influence of melatonin on reproductive health.[31] It is easy to see why melatonin may play a significant role in egg health.

Only a handful of small studies have been done on melatonin in human infertility patients. In one high-quality study, women who received 3 mg of melatonin had a greater number of mature eggs and higher-grade embryos than women who received a placebo.[32] An analysis of several small studies also found that melatonin treatment significantly increased the number of eggs retrieved and the amount of good-quality embryos.[33] One study showed that egg quality improved when melatonin was taken along with myoinositol and folic acid in women undergoing IVF, especially in women with PCOS.[34]

The dose of melatonin taken to support sleep is 0.3 mg to 1 mg. However, there is debate about the most appropriate dose for improvement in fertility. A dose of more than 3 mg may result in adverse side effects, including headaches, dizziness, nausea, and daytime drowsiness. When it comes to melatonin, a little goes a long way—so aim for sweet dreams, not a daytime snooze-fest. And melatonin can have significant interactions with many common drugs, so if you are going to start taking it, discuss it with your physician.

Though more studies are needed, melatonin may be helpful as a supplement to improve egg quality and quantity, working behind the scenes to protect and support reproductive health.

DHEA

You may have heard about the supplement DHEA (dehydroepiandrosterone), particularly for women with diminished ovarian reserve. All hormones your body produces start as cholesterol and go through multiple pathways, being modified by various enzymes, before reaching their final form. Like Legos, the same building blocks can turn into wildly different creations with very different purposes and functions depending on how they are assembled. DHEA is one of these precursor hormones. It is the building block for androgens (male hormones) such as testosterone, but women's bodies produce it too. And it occurs naturally in wild yam and soy.[35]

Though DHEA has some androgenic activity itself—its potential side effects can include acne, skin changes, and unwanted hair—it is unclear exactly how DHEA works within the body.[36] There is some evidence that specific markers for ovarian aging may improve after using DHEA, which suggests that it impacts egg health directly.[37] Another small study zeroed in on DHEA's impact on mitochondrial function and energy use, suggesting that it improves egg function.[38] A few small studies have tried to evaluate the impact of DHEA on ovarian reserve testing, including AMH, FSH, and antral follicle count, with conflicting results.[39] In the IVF world, what we care most about is IVF outcomes. But the studies that have been done on this also had only small numbers of participants and showed mixed outcomes.[40] A meta-analysis, which combined several studies and reanalyzed their data, showed that DHEA did not impact individual parts of the process, such as egg retrieval, implantation, or miscarriage. And when only the highest quality studies were analyzed, there was no improvement in the clinical pregnancy rates.[41] So although DHEA has shown some promise in improving egg and mitochondrial function, the mixed and inconclusive results from research so far limit its current role in fertility treatment.

MYOINOSITOL

Myoinositol plays an important role in cell signaling, cell formation, and growth. It also helps protect against oxidative stress.[42] One of its key functions is in insulin metabolism, something frequently impaired in women who do not regularly ovulate.[43] There it helps to improve the insulin signaling system, which is vital to a wide variety of functions within the cell.

Myoinositol is a type of inositol, a sugar that is made in the body. The other primary inositol in the body is D-chiroinositol. Myoinositols help encourage estrogen production, while D-chiroinositols impair it. In a study examining relative concentrations of each type of inositol, the best ratio for fertility patients was found to be 40 parts of myoinositol to 1 part D-chiroinositol.[44] In the world of inositols, myoinositol takes the lead, while D-chiroinositol plays a supportive role — because fertility is all about teamwork!

Inositols have shown a positive impact on insulin-to-bloodsugar ratios and menstrual cycle regularity, as well as a suppressive effect on LH, prolactin, testosterone, and insulin.[45] This is especially relevant to fertility patients because hyperinsulinemia (high blood insulin levels) impacts up to 80 percent of PCOS patients, and PCOS with hyperinsulinemia occurs in 15–20 percent of infertile women.[46] Several research groups have analyzed myo-inositol's impact on women with PCOS. Though one study did not show any improvement in pregnancy rates, multiple other studies found improved pregnancy rates when myoinositol was compared to metformin or a placebo.[47]

Though the data is not conclusive, inositols do appear to be the multitaskers of the fertility world — helping to balance insulin, regulate cycles, and even boost pregnancy rates, especially in women with PCOS. Myoinositol might just be the unsung hero your ovaries have been waiting for!

WHAT ABOUT THE SWIMMERS?

We would be remiss not to mention supplements that may improve sperm production and function. Though we often rely on intracytoplasmic sperm injection when we are dealing with abnormal sperm profiles, every embryologist would much rather have the opportunity to pick the ideal sperm from hundreds, thousands, or even millions than having to choose the best option from a very small number. Anything we can do to improve sperm parameters has the potential to improve outcomes.

Free radicals can play havoc with sperm, just as they can with any other cell. Their negative effects on sperm may be increased by extreme temperatures, alcohol consumption, obesity, and nutritional deficiencies. Semen naturally carries antioxidants to protect sperm function. So it makes sense that antioxidant supplements could be beneficial.

Vitamin A (in the form of retinoic acid) is important to the development of baby spermatids into mature active sperm. It also initiates the process of dividing DNA correctly.[48] Vitamin C, normally found within semen, prevents DNA damage within the sperm. Vitamin E neutralizes free radicals and boosts other antioxidants. One study evaluating the effects of vitamin C and vitamin E supplementation over two months showed an improved ICSI success rate in patients with DNA damage. Another study examined men with low sperm motility and poor morphology who were given either vitamin E and selenium or a placebo. Those who received vitamin E and selenium saw improvements in motility and morphology, with increased spontaneous pregnancy rates.[49]

Carnitines (L-carnitine and L-acetyl carnitine) provide energy for sperm and are involved in sperm maturation and motility.[50] L-carnitine is a substance required for human metabolism. It's so important in sperm health that L-carnitine levels are two thousand times higher in the epididymis (the tubules where sperm mature and are stored until ejaculation) than in the blood.[51] Recent studies have provided good evidence that carnitine supplementation can lead to improvement in sperm velocity, count, concentration, and motility.[52] You can think of carnitines as rocket fuel for sperm, powering them up for speed, strength, and the ultimate mission.

N-acetylcysteine (NAC) helps to replenish glutathione, a powerful antioxidant in the body that protects cells, including sperm, from damage caused by free radicals and toxins. There is some evidence that NAC, when taken for at least three months, can improve sperm shape and decrease DNA fragmentation. Additionally, hormonal profiles (FSH, LH, and testosterone, all of which are essential to sperm production) may improve.[53]

Melatonin may be helpful for male partners too, by reducing free radical damage in the testes and improving sperm function. Melatonin reduces mitochondrial DNA damage in sperm and improves the proliferation of testicular stem cells, enhancing sperm production.[54]

The multitude of supplements that potentially enhance IVF outcomes grows as more research is completed year after year. From antioxidants like CoQ10 and melatonin, which combat oxidative stress, to vitamins and minerals, which support overall reproductive health, the potential benefits are promising. The world of fertility supplements is like a buffet — there are so many tempting options. But it's best to pick wisely with your REI specialist as your guide. After all, when it comes to IVF, every little boost can feel like a step closer to making dreams come true!

PART II

The IVF Process

Key Steps on the Path to Pregnancy

CHAPTER 7

. . . .

Stimulating Success and Supercharging Egg Development

Your IVF journey is about to begin. This chapter will take some of the mystery out of what happens during your stimulation. Knowledge is power, and knowing the general course of events will make your stimulation less stressful. It is likely you will be anxious during your stimulation simply because you have so many hopes and dreams depending on the success of your cycle. That is to be expected. And with guidance from us and your IVF team, you will be one step closer to making your dream a reality.

GETTING YOUR MEDS

Your clinic orders meds in preparation for your stimulation, usually through a mail-order specialty pharmacy. These specialty pharmacies provide quality medications at a lower cost than most brick-and-mortar pharmacies. In fact, most neighborhood

> Make sure someone is at home to receive the medications or have them sent to a friend or workplace where they can be brought in out of the elements right away.

pharmacies do not carry the specific medications you will take for IVF. There are many specialty pharmacies, and you may have a choice. We generally recommend getting all your medications from one pharmacy. Having multiple pharmacies in the mix increases the odds of something getting missed. However, you may need to go through a specific supplier if you have insurance coverage for your medications. You will receive a huge box of meds from your mail-order pharmacy. When you receive them, ensure you know which ones need refrigeration and which do not. If unsure, call the pharmacy, and they can guide you.

Your first delivery likely will not contain all the medications you will need during your IVF stimulation. The initial order often contains just a limited amount — like eight or ten days' worth — to get you through the first part of the stimulation. Most stimulations last longer, and refills are necessary. Your clinical team gives you prescription refills in anticipation of this. Though having to arrange refills may seem like more work for you, it helps you avoid having leftover expensive medications in your refrigerator at the end of the cycle. So, as you are getting low on your medications, talk to your clinical team to find out how much more to order. Also, keep in mind that you need enough time to get your medications. Many mail-order pharmacies can get you medications within twenty-four hours. But you must consider weekends, holidays, season of the year, natural disasters, distance from major cities, and the unexpected (like an accidental delivery

> This may be obvious, but look all the way through the box and packing materials before throwing them out. Those vials are small and numerous.

to your next-door neighbor, who is in Jamaica for the week). It is your responsibility to make sure you have enough medications to see you through your cycle. We do not recommend waiting until your evening injection time to determine if you have enough meds. The worst call we get from a patient on a Saturday night is when we find out you did not get your trigger shot in your medication shipment. Unfortunately, as we said, most brick-and-mortar pharmacies don't stock IVF fertility medication, so in those cases, we make do with what is available.

The Art of ART (assistive reproductive technologies) MEDICATION PROTOCOLS

The weeks leading up to the actual stimulation vary from protocol to protocol. This is an area where you truly experience the art of medicine. There are several ways to prepare the ovaries to go into the stimulation. We will describe a few of the most common. However, even within the same practice, one physician may do things differently than another. This is normal. There is no one right way to do a stimulation, and many factors may play into your personal regimen, including age, ovarian reserve, the desired number of children, and insurance coverage.

The Pre-Race Warm-up

Some of the most common IVF stimulation protocols are an antagonist protocol (with or without oral contraceptive pills), an estrogen priming protocol, a microdose leuprolide (leuprolide flare) protocol, and a luteal phase (day 21) leuprolide protocol. Let's take a look at how these start.

Either the antagonist or microdose leuprolide protocols may be preceded by a period of time on oral contraceptive pills. OCPs serve a very important purpose. They help the follicles get organized and

117

create a tighter cohort — that is, they assist a group of follicles at the starting line to grow together at the same time. The largest follicles tend to call the shots, meaning these follicles determine when you are ready to trigger. If you have a good number of follicles traveling together, they will meet at the finish line at approximately the same time, thereby likely resulting in more mature eggs at the time of retrieval.

If OCPs are going to be used, they are usually taken for three to six weeks. A shorter duration increases the risk of a functional cyst, which is a large follicle that produces hormones. A longer duration may oversuppress ovarian function, preventing the expected response to the stimulation. These are guidelines; your REI specialist may do something differently based on your situation.

If you have contraindications to taking OCPs, you may have a no-OCP or natural start. These contraindications include, but are not limited to, a personal history of blood clots or clotting disorder, nicotine use over age thirty-five to forty, extreme intolerance to OCPs in the past, and, in some circumstances, poor ovarian reserve. It is normal and common to have side effects like mood swings and spotting or light bleeding while on OCPs for a short duration; these are not usually considered contraindications to OCP use.

Another protocol commonly used, especially in women with diminished ovarian reserve — something that is determined based either on age or on ovarian testing — is an estrogen priming cycle. This type of stim start can have a variety of permutations, but there are certain similarities. Ovulation is determined either by using an ovulation predictor kit (OPK) midcycle or by checking your luteal phase progesterone level, which involves drawing blood usually during cycle days 18

> The **luteal phase** is the roughly two weeks after ovulation, when progesterone increases.

through 21, depending on your average cycle length. If you use OPKs, you will start the priming process about a week later. If you use progesterone levels, priming usually begins immediately. The priming aims to let your ovaries rest and get organized so that when we start the stimulation, they are ready to party! Priming medications usually involve estrogen, which may be in the form of patches, oral medication, vaginal medication, or injectable estradiol. Some REI specialists also use a GnRH antagonist or oral GnRH agonist as part of the priming cocktail. When you start your period or reach another endpoint specified by your physician, you will call your clinic to begin your stimulation.

The oldest of these protocols is the luteal phase (day 21) leuprolide protocol. The day 21 leuprolide and leuprolide flare protocols utilize the dual nature of leuprolide (discussed in Chapter 3). When leuprolide is first administered, it stimulates follicular growth within the ovary by acting on the hypothalamus, consequently increasing FSH release from the pituitary. This FSH release augments the FSH and LH you get through gonadotropin injections to stimulate follicle growth. Later in the cycle, leuprolide prevents ovulation by suppressing LH release, so that your eggs aren't released before retrieval.

At the Starting Line

Now that we have the prep done, you are ready to start your stimulation and have your baseline appointment. At baseline, your REI specialist will do a vaginal ultrasound of your ovaries and uterus. At the beginning of the cycle, the endometrial lining in the uterus is usually thin. At this point, your ovaries are the stars of the show. We want your follicles small, ideally each less than 10 mm, and all approximately the same size. Depending on the protocol type, your REI may want you to have an estradiol level below a certain threshold, often below 80 pg/mL. If these two criteria are not met, your physician may recommend waiting to start your cycle. We know this can be extremely frustrating. If your doctor recommends continuing OCPs or waiting until another cycle, remember that they are experienced in running these cycles and want everything they can control to be perfect. It may take an extra ounce of patience, but you don't want to look back and wish you had followed their recommendations.

Running the Race

Monitoring visits at your clinic check your progress as you go through your stimulation. Exactly how these visits look varies from clinic to clinic. You may have specific appointment times, or the clinic may work on a first-come, first-served basis. Some clinics draw your labs on-site; in other cases you may need to go to a blood draw station at a commercial laboratory (and if you are using a commercial laboratory and are paying cash, often you can pay for the labs through your clinic to get a better price for the labs within your treatment cycle). You will need your labs drawn in the morning to receive same-day results. Make sure you know when the cutoff is so that you can get results back later on the same day. Your clinic needs the results by midafternoon to decide your regimen that evening. You do not need to be fasting when you go in for your blood draws, but be sure you are well hydrated, since it will make the draw easier. Also, if you live in a colder climate, staying warm will help make your veins more accessible.

In addition to monitoring your estradiol levels, which should gradually rise during your stimulation, you will have vaginal ultrasounds. These ultrasounds are scheduled every two to three days after an initial stimulation period to watch your follicles grow (the average follicle grows about 2 mm per day). Your physician, another physician in the practice, a nurse or physician assistant, or a sonographer may perform the ultrasound. These ultrasounds provide a wealth of information to your REI. We watch to see if the cohort grows in synchrony at the expected rate and if there are any signs of other things that we need to be aware of during the stimulation. We also look for the development of free fluid in the pelvis, which could be a sign of ovarian hyperstimulation syndrome, particularly nearing the end of your stimulation.

It is best to empty your bladder right before your ultrasound. A full bladder will make the ultrasound less comfortable and limit the ability to visualize the pelvis. Sometimes patients are surprised that we are doing vaginal instead of abdominal ultrasounds, but this ultrasound method gives us the best imaging of your uterus and ovaries. Also, don't worry about us if you are on your period or haven't shaved your legs. This is what we do every day!

You may receive instructions for your upcoming medication regimen at your appointment. However, it is common to receive communication from your clinic regarding your personal instructions for that evening and potentially the next few days via phone, email, or secure portal later in the day. We encourage you to make sure you understand your instructions and ask for any necessary clarification. If you are uncertain what to do next, communicate with your clinic! Even if your clinic is closed, there is someone on call to assist you. But dealing with these types of issues during regular business hours is best since you communicate with your usual team. After hours, the person on call will not have the same intimate level of knowledge regarding your specific scenario, though they are very knowledgeable about the IVF process.

As you go through your stimulation, your follicles grow. As they grow, several physical and hormonal changes occur. How you feel during this period can vary. Regarding the physical changes, knowing your baseline and how much change happens during an IVF stimulation is important. The average size of an ovary is approximately 3 cm by 1.5 cm. An average "mature" follicle will be about 2 cm in diameter. So each of your large follicles may be close to the size of your normal ovary. Feeling pressure and discomfort is expected. Stretchy pants are your friend. The more follicles you have, the more marked your symptoms may be. However, if you have severe pain, notify your physician's office immediately. Ovarian torsion — a condition where the ovary twists on its blood supply — is a rare condition that can occur as your ovary grows; that is why you'll be told to avoid vigorous activities such as running or jumping while undergoing stimulation or recovery. Also, growing those follicles takes a lot of water and energy. Stay well hydrated and get some rest. We ask a lot of your body right now, so treat it kindly. Estrogen levels also rise significantly as your eggs grow, and this can cause breast tenderness and moodiness. Some weight gain during this time is very common and expected. This generally resolves by your next period. Don't let the changes your body is experiencing distract you from the fact that completing the stimulation process is a huge accomplishment. You are a badass.

Nearing the Finish Line: The Final Push

After approximately ten to twelve days of stimulation, most women will be ready for the trigger. The trigger shot causes the eggs to mature and prepare for release. The decision to trigger is complex. Factors that your physician considers include the size of the cohort's follicles, estrogen levels, age and ovarian reserve, and any signs of impending OHSS. These factors affect not only the timing but also the medication used. Most trigger shots are administered thirty-six hours before the planned egg retrieval, but in your case it may be as early as thirty-four hours or as late as thirty-seven. The timing of this shot is *very* important. Set your alarm!

Medications used for the trigger include hCG, leuprolide, or even both (when a dual trigger is used). Physician preference and your particular clinical course dictate which you use. For details on these medications, see Chapter 3. Many clinics will do post-trigger labs or monitoring to ensure you have absorbed the medication as expected and have the appropriate physiologic response. If you did an hCG trigger or dual trigger, you may have an hCG level drawn or be advised to do a urine pregnancy test the next morning. In this situation, a positive test does not mean you are pregnant; it means that the medication has been absorbed correctly. If you do a leuprolide trigger, you may have an LH and progesterone level drawn or be asked to use an ovulation predictor kit. The LH level or OPK helps us know if your brain responded appropriately to the leuprolide, and the progesterone level lets us know if your follicles responded appropriately to your own LH. If any of these tests suggest you did not respond as expected, you may be re-triggered with a different medication or a higher dose, and your retrieval will be delayed by a day. This is rare, but a possibility.

We hope that this chapter has provided you with guidance as to what to expect during your stimulation. It can be an intense couple of weeks. However, it is a small amount of time to dedicate to making your dream come true.

. . . .

CHAPTER 8

Behind the Scenes at the Egg Retrieval: An Insider's View

The moment you have been waiting for is almost here! If you feel butterflies when you think about IVF, that's normal. Many people worry more about the outcome than about the procedure itself. IVF may feel like playing the lottery, where the odds are stacked against you, but that's not the case at all! The odds of winning the Powerball lottery are about 1 in 298 million. Your chances of having a baby may be as high as 65 percent with just a single attempt — those odds are worth taking.

This chapter covers everything you need to know about what goes on behind the scenes during egg retrieval. You will learn who will see you in the pre-op area, and who will be with you in the operating room during your procedure. You also find out what takes place throughout the procedure itself. By the end of this chapter, you will have a much better idea of all the steps you will experience the day of your egg retrieval.

PREGAME IN THE SURGERY CENTER

When you arrive at the surgery center, you meet a team of people before the procedure begins. Viewing this group as a team is a great way to think about all these medical professionals, who have many years of training and help patients through this complicated process every day. They understand that you are excited but probably nervous and will try to lessen your fears.

The Surgery Nurse

You and your support person will be brought into the surgery preoperative area. The first person you will probably meet is the nurse who will take care of you before and after surgery. They will give you information about the procedure and make sure to address all your concerns. At that time, you will receive instructions about postsurgery care, and you'll review and sign consents for the procedure if that has not been done already. You'll be given a gown to change into. The nurse will then start an IV, which will be used to give you anesthesia.

The Anesthesia Specialist

The next team member you meet will be an anesthesiologist or nurse anesthetist. Before the anesthesiologist starts the medicine to slide you into sleep, they double-check your medication and any medication allergies. They will confirm that you have not eaten or drunk any liquids over the past several hours. In addition, the anesthesiologist often asks about alcohol or drug use. These details can impact how much medicine you will need to stay sedated, so now is the time to be 100 percent truthful. These professionals literally have your life in their hands and need to know if you stopped for breakfast on the way (which is not a good idea).

Once you're in the procedure room, the anesthesiologist gives you a medication called propofol to bring on a nice nap. This medicine may sting a little bit as it goes through your IV, but it acts so fast that after a short time you won't even care. Throughout the procedure, the anesthesiologist closely monitors your breathing and blood pressure. If your heart rate becomes too fast or slow, they can use other medications for

> An **anesthesiologist** or **nurse anesthetist** is a professional with specialized training to keep patients safe and comfortable during surgery.

control. You will be sedated during the procedure but will be able to breathe on your own and will not need a breathing tube. In most cases, you won't feel or remember anything at all.

The Retrieving Doctor

The retrieving doctor will visit you before the procedure. In many programs, the doctor with whom you planned your IVF cycle may not be the person who does your egg retrieval. This is because your eggs may be ready for retrieval at any point, and physicians are not always available when that moment comes. While your REI specialist may be disappointed if they cannot be available for the egg retrieval, it is far more important that retrievals occur on the eggs' timeline, not the doctor's. Most of the time, though, it's your doctor who does perform the embryo transfer.

What to Expect Afterward

Your retrieving physician will explain how you may feel after the procedure. Most women feel lower abdominal soreness for about twenty-four hours after the egg retrieval — similar to the feeling after an intense ab workout at the gym. The blood and fluids remaining in the abdomen after the procedure can irritate the inside of the body cavity. You may even be one or two pounds heavier, but within a day you will lose that weight as your body returns to normal. Usually, those symptoms can be treated with a combination of ibuprofen, acetaminophen, and some TLC from your partner. The bloating that you felt before the procedure does not immediately go away; it gradually dissipates over the next couple of weeks. Once your menstrual cycle starts, you will begin to feel more normal.

Some women may have worsening bloating, abdominal pain, shortness of breath, or vomiting after the retrieval. If any of those symptoms occur, you should let your IVF doctor or nurse know. Call the office; you should be able to reach the staff or, if it's after hours, speak to someone on call. If your pain is more intense than you expect, it is wise to reach out to your clinic.

All patients who do IVF undergo stimulation with the aim of producing more than one egg. Most women tolerate this stimulation with minimal discomfort, as we've seen, but a few patients become moderately or severely hyperstimulated. One way to monitor for hyperstimulation is by comparing your weight and waist measurement the day before retrieval to the day after. If you gain more than five to ten pounds, or if your waist circumference is one inch (or more) larger than before, you should contact your IVF team. Depending on your case, they may bring you in for evaluation on that day or just have you continue to monitor your symptoms. If you experience significant abdominal pain, nausea, or shortness of breath (you have trouble breathing even when sitting), you should call the doctor's office, even if it is after regular business hours.

How Many Eggs Will Be Retrieved?

Finally, before the procedure your doctor may give you a ballpark idea of the anticipated number of eggs to be retrieved. Remember, your physician does not have a crystal ball, and every doc has had the experience of giving an estimate for this number but getting significantly more or fewer eggs than expected, so they may be vague on this point beforehand. Since the IV pain medicine makes you feel as if you drank a couple of strong margaritas, unexpected news that the doctor retrieved a smaller number of eggs than projected may cause a disproportionately tearful response. Your doc does not want you to head home after the procedure in that state, especially because excellent results may still emerge from small numbers. Sometimes it is just best to wait and see.

Prior to the procedure, it is impossible to know exactly how many eggs will be retrieved; the ease of accessing both ovaries for egg retrieval; or the strength of the eggs' attachment to the ovary. Also keep in mind that the egg is literally *one* cell — so small we cannot see it without magnification. We only learn an egg has actually been retrieved once the embryologist finds it in the petri dish. We know that each follicle contains one egg, but even despite excellent technique and best efforts, not all follicles will provide an egg. Fortunately, about 70 to 80 percent of the time, an egg is retrieved from a large follicle.

Next Steps

After you've met the team, it is time to give kisses and hugs to your support person. Then don't forget to empty your bladder on the way to the procedure room. If your partner needs to leave a fresh sperm sample, he will be whisked away to the collection room. Yes, he will probably be having a better time in the collection room than you will in the OR!

EGG HUNTING:
IT'S NOT JUST FOR EASTER

An IVF operating room differs from most other ORs, as embryos are very particular about their environment. They aren't fans of contaminated air, so IVF ORs usually have positive pressure systems to keep out stray particles and also have advanced filtration systems. Lighting is kept a bit lower and temperatures a bit higher to cater to the whims of your eggs and embryos. Of course, anything that touches the embryo — such as cleaning supplies, gloves, and the needle guide — must meet rigorous standards to prevent harm to your embryo.

Once inside the OR, you may be a bit uneasy at first, but the good news is that all you have to do is sleep. Don't worry, we don't operate until you are *out*. Unusually anxious patients may require more medication to calm their nerves. But never fear, the anesthesiologist always wins — usually right in the middle of a very interesting story patients start telling us but never finish.

Positive pressure systems: Air systems where the pressure inside the room is greater than the pressure outside it. This causes air to flow out rather than in whenever the door is opened, leaving the air inside as clean as possible.

The Scrub Nurse

Just before you are given anesthesia, you will meet the scrub nurse, another key member of the team. The scrub nurse hands the instruments to the doctor and, after the retrieval, passes the test tube (hence the name "test tube baby") containing the eggs to another nurse. The scrub nurse is also a whiz at putting together complicated tubing and attaching it to the suction machine and the test tube.

The Embryologist: An Eagle Eye

The embryologist may or may not come to meet you, but this professional is critical to your success. You may not have heard much about the embryologist prior to this point. In most clinics there are several embryologists, and they are the unsung heroes in any IVF program. If the physician is the quarterback of this team, embryologists are the amazing wide receivers who catch the football and run down the field to score the winning touchdown.

The embryologist receives the fluid collected from your ovary. While the operating team works in the OR, the embryology team carefully looks through the fluid for the tiny eggs — not an easy task. The embryologist makes this arduous job look simple. After finding an egg, the embryologist will transfer it to another container for safekeeping. Some embryologists may be physically present in the room, working with a mobile incubator similar to a baby incubator. Other clinics are set up with a pass-through window like the one you see in some kitchens. The nurse passes the tubes through the window, and the embryologist examines the fluid under the microscope in a different room. Embryologists then notify the team of the egg count before you go home.

Embryologists also introduce your eggs to the sperm. If that first "date" is successful, they will be the first to know, about twenty-four hours after your egg retrieval. The embryologists babysit your embryos in the lab for five to seven days until you have blastocysts. They also biopsy the embryo if you are planning to do genetic testing. (To our embryologist colleagues who may read this: We know full well you are way more than just babysitters, which is why we have dedicated several chapters to your work in this book.)

> A **blastocyst** is a mature embryo made up of 150 to 300 cells.

The Circulating Nurse

Also present in the OR will be a circulating nurse. This person takes care of anything you or the retrieving doctor needs once you are in the OR. The circulating nurse also leads the "time out" process at the start of surgery — a measure to ensure the patient's safety, confirming everyone knows all the details of your care, including what medications you are taking, your allergies, and any other important or unique issues related to your care. It is also the circulating nurse who passes the test tube containing your eggs from the scrub nurse to the embryologist.

Egg Retrieval

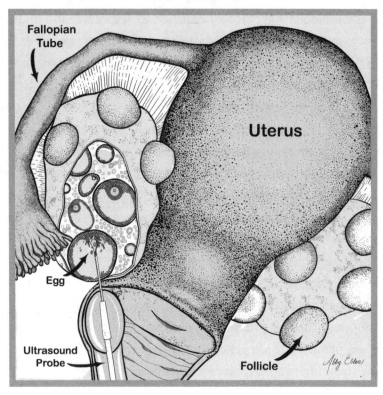

The doctor inserts a vaginal ultrasound probe and visualizes the ovary. A needle is carefully guided through the wall of the vagina and into the follicle (the fluid-filled sac containing the egg). Suction removes the fluid and egg from each accessible follicle on the ovary. The same procedure is carried out on the other side until all follicles have been aspirated.

EGG HUNTING:
THE PROCEDURE

Remember the ultrasound wand that was used to look at your ovaries? We will use an identical probe to view your ovaries during the procedure. The doctor's view will be exactly what you saw on each of your monitoring visits. At this point, however, a guide for the retrieval needle attaches to the top of the ultrasound probe.

132

The needle goes through an opening in the needle guide above the ultrasound probe.

The doctor cleans your vagina with water or a nontoxic cleanser (eggs do not like soap). You receive an antibiotic through your IV to make sure that any pesky bacteria won't cause an infection. The doctor then places the ultrasound probe in your vagina. By this point in the process, your ovaries have dropped to the lowest point in your pelvis. Normally the size of limes, they are now the size of oranges or even grapefruits and should be just to the right and left of your vaginal wall. We use a twelve-inch needle to access the ovaries. This may sound long, but your ovaries are far away, and it allows us to harvest those bashful eggs. You'll be relieved to hear that the width of the needle is very thin — about the same as a needle used for giving blood.

The needle travels through the needle guide, through the wall of the vagina, into the ovary, and into a follicle. It individually pierces each follicle, aspirating (or sucking out) the fluid, which then causes the follicle to collapse. If the embryologist cannot find an egg in the initial fluid, the doctor rotates the needle 360 degrees and slowly withdraws it. At times, the doc may even put fluid back in the follicle and try again to get the stubborn egg out, a process known as "flushing." No one is more disappointed than your doc if the egg still does not emerge, but it is impossible to know why this occasionally happens. Sometimes our "egg whisperer" tricks work, and sometimes they don't!

During the procedure your doctor carefully avoids structures other than your ovary. Egg retrievals are very safe, with less than a 1 percent rate of complications, but they are still surgical procedures with risks. Such risks include injury to blood vessels, your bowel, or your bladder. If you feel significantly dizzy or have a fever after your procedure, please call immediately. If you are like the average patient, however, you will be watching Netflix and catching some Z's at home following your retrieval.

IMMEDIATELY AFTER THE PROCEDURE

After the procedure, which takes about forty-five minutes, you return to the recovery area and reunite with the first nurse you met before entering the OR. Patients feel sleepy and may tell funny stories, but rest assured that what happens at the surgery center stays at the surgery center! Nurses monitor your pulse and blood pressure, then reunite you with your support person, who will take you home. Since you have just had surgery, legally we cannot let you leave with a stranger, such as an Uber driver. Both your level of consciousness and your decision-making skills may be impaired after the procedure.

As you wake up, the nurse will see if you tolerate liquids. Even though you may have been ravenous before the procedure, your appetite will be strangely dulled. Once you can walk, the nurse will have you go to the restroom to empty your bladder. The impact of anesthesia can sometimes cause bladders to go on strike and not do their job; if this happens, you can rest and try again later. If you are still unsuccessful on the next attempt, try turning on the faucet — the sound of running water usually does the trick.

Finally, the embryologist or your physician will let you know how many eggs were retrieved. Hopefully it will be good news. If it is fewer eggs than expected, all is not lost. Remember, you need only one good egg to get pregnant.

Before you leave the clinic, you will receive additional information about the timing of fertilization and embryo development. And the staff will let you know when to expect updates on the growth of your embryo and genetic testing results. At that point you are ready to head home.

AFTER YOU GET HOME

You spend about three hours of your day with us in the surgery center. For the remainder of the day, it is best to rest. (And no chores for at least a month! Okay, that's a bit of an exaggeration, but if your partner buys it, good for you!)

Your doctor will recommend that you take pain medications (usually over-the-counter medications) for the first twenty-four hours after retrieval. Heating pads also help ease cramping. Once you head home, you can slowly start eating again. When you feel hungry, start with bland foods: think bananas and rice, not Nashville hot chicken.

You may want to consider taking the day after the procedure off from work. Remember the part about your ovaries being the size of grapefruits? If you go to work the next day and move around as normal, you will feel the still-enlarged ovaries pushing against your bowels and abdominal wall. It will feel something like having size 8 feet but walking around all day in size 5 shoes — not pleasant. After the first twenty-four hours, you should start to feel better. Your ovaries gradually decrease in size, but it may still take several weeks for them to get back to normal.

Even though you will feel much better a few days after retrieval, your ovaries are not ready to go out for a jog or head to a yoga or Pilates class. They have been through quite an ordeal and need a little downtime. Because the ovaries are so enlarged, they are more likely to twist upon themselves, cutting off their blood supply and causing severe pain; if this happens, it is an emergency, and you will need surgery to fix the problem. Ovarian torsion is rare, but we want to minimize the risk for you. That's the reason we do not want you to hit the gym or have sex until your ovaries return to normal. By the time your next menstrual cycle starts, your ovaries will have decreased in size, and it is probably safe for you to exercise, but check with your doctor first.

Over the course of the next seven days, you will hear updates about embryo development. If you opted for genetic testing on your embryos, results will come back in about three or four weeks, depending on the type of testing you are having done.

And that's it. Now you have seen inside the surgery center on the day of egg retrieval. You know the roles of all the medical professionals caring for you: the nurses, the anesthesiologist, the retrieving doctor, and the embryologist. You have also learned how the procedure is performed. When your menstrual cycle starts, you may be able to begin medications for the next phase, the frozen embryo transfer; if you do a fresh embryo transfer instead, you will return just a few days after the egg retrieval. Choosing between fresh and frozen embryo transfer is the topic of the next chapter.

CHAPTER 9

. . . .

Embryo Transfers:
Fresh Start or
Ice-Cold Surprise

There are many points in life at which fresh versus frozen is a
crucial decision. Pizza is a prime example. But it also applies to
some of the important biology in our lives. Frozen embryo transfer
(FET) has emerged as one of the most effective ways to optimize
an embryo transfer cycle. This section discusses the physiology and
medicine of retrieval cycles, transfer cycles, genetic testing, uterine
preparation, and family planning, providing a beautiful example
of the complexity of reproductive medicine. Buckle up; here we go.

DEFINITIONS

First, let's review briefly the difference between fresh embryo transfers and frozen embryo transfers. A *fresh* transfer moves immediately from egg retrieval to embryo transfer within the same
cycle, never freezing the embryo in the interim. A *frozen* embryo

transfer separates the retrieval and transfer cycles by at least a month, allowing the body to reset itself after the hormonal manipulation involved in a retrieval cycle. The embryo must be frozen between these two cycles to ensure survival — we cannot just let it languish in its dish.

THE BACKSTORY

Next, let's talk about the history of fresh versus frozen embryo transfers and why historically fresh transfers were preferred. Retrievals and fresh embryo transfers were originally done sequentially because embryo freezing technology was in its infancy and wasn't exceptionally safe for the embryos. As a result, freezing an embryo compromised the overall success of the cycle. Initially, freezing embryos was a slow process. It took quite some time for an embryo to drop from normal body temperature to North Pole levels. The time it took to slowly drop the temperature provided more opportunity for ice crystals to form within the embryo. Ice crystals are fabulous in a snow cone on a hot summer day, but they are tiny little chaos goblins inside an embryo.

Then along came a process called vitrification. Vitrification is a fast-freeze process. In vitrification, the embryo is essentially dehydrated and cooled down so quickly that ice crystals do not have the opportunity to form. When ice crystals don't develop, the embryo's integrity remains intact, and you have a much healthier embryo at the time of thaw. This was a monumental change to the game because it meant we no longer felt obligated to cram both embryo creation and embryo transfer into the same cycle for the benefit of embryo integrity. As a result, doctors and patients could choose the best option instead of being forced into a one-size-fits-all pathway.

WHY FRESH EMBRYO TRANSFERS ARE NOT IDEAL

. . . .

If you are interested in getting into the scientific weeds, this section is for you. If not, you can skip it and move on to the practical aspects of fresh versus frozen embryo transfer.

Two processes in human reproduction are highly time-dependent. The first is ovulation and the second is endometrial priming, called decidualization. Ovulation is triggered by a spontaneous LH surge during normal reproduction or by a trigger shot in an IVF cycle. The timing of the trigger shot is critical for optimal egg maturity and the ability to extract eggs after they've matured while still in the ovary. During the first half of the cycle, the endometrium is exposed to estrogen. Estrogen exposure must be long and high enough to turn the endometrium into a cushy landing pad for the embryo. The second important process, decidualization, primes the endometrium to aid embryo implantation. Decidualization depends on the timing of progesterone secretion and creates a precise time for implantation, known as the window of implantation.

These time-dependent processes start with the growing egg. While the egg grows, its surrounding cells produce estrogen. Once the egg ovulates, its former housing unit, the follicle, is not abandoned; it transforms from an egg house into a hormone factory. This hormone factory is called a corpus luteum. The cells previously producing only estrogen change and begin to produce progesterone, priming the uterine lining for implantation. Progesterone secretion too early or too late impairs implantation. The body naturally ties progesterone production to ovulation so that progesterone is secreted at the perfect time.

During a natural cycle, progesterone is unlikely to rise prematurely. During a fresh stimulation cycle, however, progesterone may increase several days before egg retrieval, thereby impairing the precise timing needed to prepare the endometrium. With a fresh transfer cycle, the timing of the trigger and endometrial preparation often are out of sync due to altered hormone levels during IVF.

Until the last decade, fertility doctors asked patients to take the final trigger injection when three of the most prominent follicles were around 18 mm in diameter. At that point, estrogen levels were high, but progesterone levels were still low. Doctors had a good chance of getting mature eggs before premature progesterone exposure irreparably changed the uterine lining. The downside is that we would leave behind many small and midsize follicles that could have produced mature eggs if we had waited longer to trigger.

Hormone levels in fresh retrieval cycles are spectacularly different from those during a natural cycle, when usually just a single egg is released. In a fresh retrieval cycle, hormones are pumped out at exponentially higher levels than usual. We are trying to grow as many eggs as possible, and each one produces estrogen and later progesterone. That results in hormone levels much higher than normal physiologic levels and may impact implantation rates in a fresh transfer.

To summarize, high hormone levels are awesome and desired, but they cause problems for a successful fresh transfer. High estrogen levels and rising progesterone levels after ovarian stimulation and trigger often negatively impact a fresh transfer just five days later. Conversely, in frozen embryo transfer cycles, hormonal exposure and timing are tightly controlled and not nearly as problematic. By doing each procedure separately, we can optimize success rates for both.

The timing of an embryo transfer and the subsequent success rates are highly dependent on how long the uterine lining has been exposed to progesterone. Progesterone is a magical hormone that allows for the implantation process to occur. No baby happens without it. As such, you need to nail it regarding exposure hours. There's something called a window of implantation, which is the sweet spot for transferring the embryo after progesterone exposure. Too soon or too late and the whole party is ruined. If you're doing a fresh transfer cycle, it is more likely that progesterone will increase prematurely. This premature increase disrupts the carefully orchestrated dance between ovulation and implantation. Essentially, the timing of the endometrium and the stage of the embryo may not be in sync, which can negatively affect your chances of pregnancy success. FET cycles cleanly separate hormone events that occur in ovulation from those that occur in implantation so that the embryo and lining are in step with each other.

Studies examining fresh versus frozen transfers show good frozen embryo success rates in patients receiving appropriately timed, consistent, adequate amounts of progesterone. The studies using effective doses of progesterone before transfer typically show frozen embryo transfer being the more successful option.[1] In studies showing that fresh transfers might be better, a significant potential reason is that there may have been suboptimal dosing of progesterone during the frozen cycles that were studied; as a result, the progesterone in the fresh cycle did the job better, therefore winning out in terms of success rates. The types of progesterone that result in excellent success rates for FET vary (we cover this in Chapter 13).

When you're trying to fit both egg retrieval and embryo transfer together in a single cycle, you must compromise, taking into consideration hormone levels and follicle size. Compromise is a fantastic technique in a relationship, but not in the embryology lab, where we want the best of every scenario. So as a result, we have started to separate out egg retrievals and frozen transfers.

DREAMS ON ICE: ADVANTAGES TO FET

Although most transfers are designed to be done with frozen embryos because the success rates are better, there are times in which a frozen embryo transfer is the only reasonable option available, such as when we are trying to avoid ovarian hyperstimulation syndrome or doing genetic testing.

Avoiding Ovarian Hyperstimulation Syndrome

Frozen embryo transfer is one of the best ways to avoid OHSS because it removes the possibility of an immediate pregnancy that may dangerously worsen the disease. We've mentioned OHSS before, and Chapter 12 gives you all the nitty-gritty details, but for now it's enough to say that it is more likely to occur with a prolonged presence of the pregnancy hormone hCG. The ability to do frozen transfers has opened the possibility of stimulating you longer and more aggressively with medication to get more eggs without increasing the likelihood of severe OHSS.

One reason FET reduces your chances of developing OHSS is that it removes the presence of hCG produced by a pregnancy, since you won't get pregnant immediately. The other reason you are less likely to get OHSS is that with FET a leuprolide trigger may be used to mature the eggs. Using an hCG trigger can set the wheels in motion for OHSS. Leuprolide triggers are helpful because they allow us to avoid an hCG trigger while still getting good maturity in the resulting eggs. Leuprolide also shuts down the pituitary. This means that the organ making the hormones perpetuating hyperstimulation syndrome is completely shut down. Estrogen levels drop, leading to faster resolution of the symptoms. You are safer, and it shortens the duration of symptoms. However, leuprolide triggers negatively affect the endometrium, and subsequent embryo transfer in that cycle is not recommended.

Performing Advanced Genetic Testing

Another time when frozen embryo transfer becomes mandatory is when advanced genetic testing is done on the embryos. Back in the olden days (when, of course, embryologists had to walk to the lab in the snow uphill both ways), genetic testing was rudimentary. These details are explored more in Chapter 11, but the short story starts with a biopsy of day 3 embryos and seeing the results of that rudimentary genetic testing the next day, providing only a snippet of genetic information regarding whether it was safe to transfer the embryos or not. Now, instead of looking at a measly few pieces of DNA on a couple of chromosomes, up to the entire genome is sequenced by taking a few cells from a blastocyst (a day 5 to 7 embryo). Understandably, such sequencing is not a quick, overnight process. It generally takes several weeks to get the high-quality, detailed information available from modern genetic testing, and this is impossible with a fresh transfer. At the point of blastocyst biopsy, the embryo is fully mature and cannot survive much longer outside the uterus. We must preserve its integrity, so into the freezer it goes.

WHEN LESS IS ACTUALLY MORE: ELECTIVE SINGLE EMBRYO TRANSFER

Freezing technology revolutionized the number of embryos that we transfer safely and efficaciously. With older, less developed freezing technology, both patients and physicians wanted to transfer multiple embryos at one time in order to increase success rates. At that time, freezing techniques led to poorer-quality embryos as compared to fresh embryos, with less chance of resulting in a successful pregnancy. Now that we freeze embryos without impacting safety or efficacy, we can leave them cryopreserved for as long as we want. To our knowledge, there is no known point when freezer storage becomes too long. (Fun fact: The longest-frozen embryo that resulted in a pregnancy was thirty years old!) This allows us to transfer one embryo at a time because we know that we can go back and prepare the uterus as many times as we need to get a pregnancy and have a great chance of success. This maximizes the chance of you and your baby having a safe and uneventful pregnancy and delivery.

Perfecting the technique of frozen embryo transfer keeps you safe by avoiding multi-fetal pregnancies, thereby averting the many complications multiple babies bring, such as hyperemesis gravidarum (lots of vomiting during pregnancy), premature delivery, gestational diabetes, gestational hypertension, and preeclampsia. It protects the baby from complications of prematurity, including difficulty breathing, difficulty feeding, intellectual disability, a stay in the neonatal intensive care unit, and a host of other problems.

For many years, IVF had a bad but well-deserved rap for providing the world (and reality TV shows) with triplets, quadruplets, or more. Now, IVF is the fertility procedure most likely to result in a singleton pregnancy because we usually transfer only one embryo at a time. We tell all our patients that single embryo transfer is best. We do not want them on the cover of *Time* magazine or with their own reality show after delivering a dozen babies at once. The rate of multiple gestation with IVF differs greatly compared to an insemination cycle, where the twin rate is often 5 to 8 percent because the sperm fertilize the multiple eggs released. With single embryo transfer, the only twins that occur are identical ones, where the embryo splits into two early in development, after implantation. The identical twin rate with a single embryo transfer is approximately 1.5 percent, which is about what you encounter with naturally conceived pregnancies.

WHEN THE STARS ALIGN: PERFECT CONDITIONS FOR A FRESH EMBRYO TRANSFER

While frozen embryo transfers have generally become the rule, rules were made to be broken. In medicine, the words "always" or "never" rarely apply, and that holds true for fresh and frozen transfers. That said, the stars must be neatly aligned before the benefit of a fresh transfer outweighs the success of doing a frozen transfer. Let's review the circumstances needed to make a fresh transfer a good idea.

No Preimplantation Genetic Testing

For patients wanting a fresh transfer, preimplantation genetic testing is not an option. It takes too long to receive PGT results to complete a fresh transfer. However, you can do it on any extra embryos not getting transferred in that specific cycle.

Transfer or Bust

Some patients want a transfer regardless of the embryo quality, for ethical, moral, religious, or other personal reasons. Another reason is that some people want to minimize any manipulation of their embryo(s). This may translate to the transfer of an embryo with questionable quality. When a poor-quality embryo is frozen, the chances that it will survive the freezing and thawing process decrease. Some people have such poor-quality embryos that they do not even survive in culture to the blastocyst stage. While we think damage caused by freezing is minimal (as evidenced by higher success rates using frozen embryos), even minimal damage can further knock down an already impaired embryo. This is particularly true in patients with poor ovarian reserve or significantly advanced reproductive age. However, in most cases, if the embryo is not a good-quality blastocyst, the transfer is not likely to result in a viable pregnancy.

Hormonal Perfection

Hormone levels during the retrieval cycle are integral to your chances of success with a fresh transfer. Naturally occurring progesterone levels and other medications may interfere with the timing of decidualization (endometrial priming), which is initiated with the first progesterone exposure. This means the follicles must be triggered before progesterone levels elevate. Premature progesterone elevation (before the trigger) often happens in older women or those with diminished ovarian reserve, making them less ideal candidates.

Medications, including GnRH agonist triggers such as leuprolide, also interfere with the endometrium. This potentially impacts many groups of patients, especially young women and those with PCOS, who have a higher risk of hyperstimulation syndrome (see Chapter 12). GnRH agonists produce an LH surge but impair endometrial receptivity by shortening the luteal phase and by altering hormone dynamics and gene expression. These changes thereby decrease the success rates for fresh embryo transfers.

Fresh transfers are often accompanied by less aggressive stimulations. In this case, "aggressive" means higher doses of medications with the intent to get as many follicles and eggs as possible. High numbers of follicles produce levels of estrogen that are high above physiologic levels (that is, the levels found in a healthy body that is functioning normally) and which are potentially hostile to a developing embryo. This environment is dissimilar to a naturally occurring cycle and is likely a reason for impaired success rates. However, if you have a less aggressive stimulation with lower estrogen levels and follicle numbers, you may be a better candidate for fresh transfer.

THE OTHER SIDE OF THE COIN

Nothing is perfect all the time. Both fresh and frozen transfers have their respective risks.

Risks of Frozen Transfers

Programmed frozen embryo transfer cycles using estrogen and progesterone supplementation are associated with an increased risk of blood pressure disorders in pregnancy such as gestational hypertension and preeclampsia.[2] It's possible different transfer protocols may decrease this risk, but it is worth considering as you make decisions.[3] Chapter 13 reviews transfer protocols in detail.

Risks of Fresh Transfers

Fresh embryo transfers frequently compromise success because of the need to juxtapose egg retrieval and endometrial preparation. During egg retrieval estrogen and progesterone levels and their effect on the endometrium are not physiologic, and the impact shows up in poorer success rates. The pressure to transfer multiple embryos, thereby increasing the risk of a multiple pregnancy, is higher in a fresh transfer due to the last-minute desire to avoid any embryo freezing. Every REI specialist has heard, "Can't you just put them both in, Doc?" at the time of a fresh transfer, only to see the havoc multiple babies wreak during a pregnancy. OHSS risks increase substantially with a fresh transfer due to the combination of recent ovarian stimulation, the required hCG trigger, and the prolonged presence of hCG with a pregnancy. Most of the really frightening and dangerous cases of OHSS arise after a fresh transfer. There is also the question of the negative impact on birth weight. Weights of babies born after fresh transfer are consistently lower than those of babies born via unassisted conception or frozen embryo transfer.[4] It is not a huge difference, less than half a pound, but the consistency of this outcome brings up the possibility of a compromised uterine environment during a fresh transfer.

Above all, talk to your doctor. The decision regarding fresh versus frozen transfer can be clear-cut, but in more complex cases, subtle nuances influence the final choice. Your physician has concrete reasons for specific recommendations and has spent a lot of time studying the data for this decision, which massively impacts success.

CHAPTER 10

. . . .

IVF:
It's a Numbers Game

*W*hat happened to all my eggs?
After egg retrieval, the quantity of embryos changes rapidly and continually. You may start with many follicles visible on your ultrasound, and that number is whittled down to far fewer actual embryos for potential transfer. That's a good thing, because the selection process may take care of itself as abnormal embryos that would never result in a pregnancy stop progressing, leaving only the heartier embryos. But, it can be a bit jarring when you learn that your twenty eggs have made only two chromosomally normal embryos. So why the big change in numbers?

Going through the stimulation process, you probably watched how your hormone levels rose, and you listened during ultrasound exams as each of your follicles was measured. You may have tried to figure out how these bits of information might translate into how many eggs you might get on retrieval day. The numbers may sound like gobbledygook to some people, but they indicate to your doc what is happening and when we should give the trigger. It is unusual for the number of follicles seen on ultrasound to equal precisely the number of eggs retrieved. There are a few reasons for this:

- Not every follicle seen on ultrasound yields an egg because some are too small and have not gone through the full process that is required to yield a releasable, mature egg. For one thing, a follicle that is 10 mm is just above the cutoff point for even being measured, much less yielding a mature egg, yet it still is counted during the scans. For another, sometimes cysts masquerade as growing follicles. A cyst may be an endometrioma with a misleading appearance that looks like a normal follicle despite being filled with endometriotic fluid. Other cysts may respond to medication and grow but won't have an egg.
- Age plays a role in this as well. Often, women in their forties have more empty follicles. As a result, we never retrieve an egg from those follicles.
- And, of course, there is the complexity of ultrasonography. Counting and measuring a 3D follicle while being able to look at it in only two dimensions is not easy. Getting accurate numbers is particularly tricky when there are many follicles to count.

FERTILIZATION: WHEN DOES THE BLIND DATE START?

After your doc aspirates eggs from the follicles, the lab work begins. Typically, the egg passes through the needle and tubing into a small test tube. As soon as the test tube is full of fluid, it's passed off to the embryologist. When the embryologist receives the tube, the fluid is placed into a petri dish, and the embryologist hunts for individual eggs. This is done under a microscope, as the diameter of the egg at this point is quite small, approximately the width of a human hair. In the lab, airflow, temperature, pH, humidity, and lighting are maintained at levels tailored to the needs

> **Embryologists** are laboratory professionals who specialize in the care and treatment of eggs, sperm, and embryos.

of the eggs. Once the eggs have been located, a process called stripping begins. First, cumulus cells (specialized cells surrounding the egg) are peeled away, either manually, enzymatically, or both. Once the clothes are off, so to speak, the remaining oocyte (egg) is evaluated with a critical eye. Oocytes generally fall into one of three categories at this point.

- The first category is a *germinal vesicle*. These eggs are like toddlers: cute to look at but not useful. They are far too immature to have any hope of accepting a sperm, successfully being fertilized, and developing into an embryo (at least with current technology). They are promptly discarded in most circumstances. These eggs usually come from small follicles or when the trigger medication did not work as expected.

- The second group, or the eggs in *metaphase I* (MI), have undergone the first metaphase of meiosis but not yet the second one (recall that meiosis is the process by which half the cell's chromosomes are removed, preparing the egg to receive a new set of chromosomes from the sperm). This grouping of eggs can be thought of as teenagers: some will mature and become productive members of society, while others won't. But, like teenagers, they may need some time to mature. With MIs, the embryologist completes the initial assessment and then looks at them again a few hours later when it's time for insemination, hoping they grew up and matured while sitting in the lab.

- The next set of eggs are mature eggs, also known as MIIs. These eggs have undergone the second metaphase of meiosis and are fully mature. These are the adults of the group. They combine with sperm in the hope of turning into a mature blastocyst down the line. Like adults, there's no guarantee they will eventually turn into a success, but the odds are much higher because they have already traveled further through the process.

Occasionally there will be an exception to these three categories, an egg with an empty zona — that is, the egg's outer layer is present but there is nothing in it. Or there may be an egg with a broken zona, where the egg fractured and is unusable. It's also possible for an egg to degenerate to the point where it falls apart before the opportunity for fertilization.

Once the eggs have been cleaned and the MIs and MIIs identified, the insemination process starts. Generally, there are two ways to accomplish fertilization: conventional insemination and intracytoplasmic sperm injection.

SPERM DETOUR

Let's detour for a minute and talk about sperm. Traditionally, sperm collection occurs by ejaculation on the day of egg retrieval, usually after two to five days of abstinence. This process allows for sperm collection at the same time as egg retrieval. Same-day collection occurs for most people, but there are some circumstances in which sperm needs to be collected at another time. One situation is when a male partner is out of town at the time of egg retrieval or must leave unexpectedly. Also, sperm providers living in another state or country frequently need to have their sperm cryopreserved due to travel logistics. Furthermore, donors virtually always have their sperm cryopreserved due to the need to carry out testing for infectious disease before usage. And last, "stage fright" occasionally occurs when the pressure to produce a sperm sample directly works against the ability to produce that sample. It is no secret that infertility negatively impacts many patients' libidos, and that applies equally to both men and women. While fresh sperm collection is a standard operating procedure in many clinics, when that is not possible, sperm cryopreservation helps work through these problems.

Unfortunately, sperm counts have steadily declined across the population in the past fifty years.[1] Occasionally, sperm numbers in the ejaculate collected on the day of egg retrieval are so small as to be unreliable, and a frozen backup specimen is required as a safety net. It is important to note that safety nets can be helpful, but they are not able to prevent all possible catastrophic scenarios. For instance, a sample with a nearly undetectable sperm count may not freeze with enough surviving sperm to be useful for even an IVF cycle. Appropriate expectations of what goes into the vial and how that relates to what comes out of the vial are vital to ensure success and avoid deeply unpleasant surprises. It is well known that the viability, motility, and appearance of sperm will decrease due to cryopreservation. Fortunately, success rates with IVF remain the same regardless of whether the sperm was previously frozen or not.[2]

The need for surgical sperm extraction emerges in men who cannot produce ejaculate containing viable sperm (a condition called azoospermia). These extractions typically are done by a reproductive urologist in the same facility as the embryology lab. These procedures are best suited for men who are azoospermic because of blockages caused by prior surgeries, such as vasectomies or failed vasectomy reversals. Men who cannot produce ejaculate with viable sperm for reasons other than blockage can also benefit from surgical sperm extraction, but success is less consistent.

For most men, a two- to five-day abstinence period has been recommended, with the goal of maximizing the quality and quantity of sperm. However, this protocol has been evolving in recent years. We know that DNA damage and fragmentation of sperm occur outside the testes, suggesting that it's better if the sperm spends less time in the epididymis. In some clinical situations, men are now told to ejaculate multiple times during the twenty-four hours leading up to retrieval, in order to get the best-quality sperm available. A new study suggests that frequent ejaculation leading up to the retrieval benefits ultimate embryo creation more than a prolonged abstinence period.[3] The fact that we don't need a large number of sperm to complete an IVF cycle makes quality over quantity a reasonable goal.

The process of sperm extraction differs based on need. Sperm can be extracted from the testes or the epididymis. This is often done with a fine needle through the scrotal skin (done after numbing the area, of course). Sometimes, more traditional surgery is used, when the scrotum and testes are surgically opened to visibly identify areas of sperm production. Many urologists are comfortable performing basic sperm aspiration procedures, but typically only urologists specializing in male fertility perform the more advanced sperm collection procedures. Fortunately, it has been shown that IVF success rates using fresh or frozen sperm were not different based on whether the sperm was extracted from the epididymis or from the testes.[4]

During the testing process, and especially when there's a low sperm count (oligospermia) or a total absence of sperm (azoospermia), a man's levels of hormones like FSH and LH may need to be checked. FSH levels indicate how effectively the signaling system works in a man, very similarly to how the system works in women. Low to normal levels of FSH demonstrate the testicles can respond to the brain's instructions. In contrast, high levels of FSH indicate that the testicles are ignoring the brain's instructions and that the brain is essentially "yelling" at the testicles to start sperm production. These levels can also indicate the effectiveness of medication in increasing sperm production. Medications typically do not help with low sperm counts due to a blockage, as presence of a blockage does not affect sperm production. Medications are more likely to be helpful when used in patients with low baseline levels of FSH and azoospermia or severe oligospermia that is due to reasons other than blockage.[5]

Several medications may potentially increase sperm production. These medications fall into two general groups: those that can be delivered as pills and those that must be delivered by injection. Injectable medications work to replicate the instructions to the testicles. As we discussed in earlier chapters, hCG can be used to replicate LH activity because of the very similar structures of these two substances. Injections of FSH may also directly duplicate instructions issued by the brain. These injectable medications can be taken one or more times a week to give consistent instructions to the testicles, maximizing sperm production. The oral medications clomiphene or anastrozole work by either altering enzyme effectiveness or decreasing estrogen levels (yes, men have estrogen too) to trick the brain into producing more FSH and LH on its own. Patients take these medications either daily or every other day. Typically a minimum of seventy-two days is required before meaningful increases in sperm count may occur, but often it takes longer.

Every discussion of medications includes review of potential adverse effects. In general, medications to increase sperm counts are safe and well tolerated. Patients with long-term exposure to high levels of FSH may see increased bone breakdown and immunological, heart, and metabolic effects, but more data is needed to see how these preliminary studies apply in the fertility setting.[6] Effects from hCG injections mimic the effects of testosterone, with high blood pressure, hair loss, acne, and a potential increase in estrogen leading to breast development.[7] Side effects from clomiphene may include headache, mood changes, dizziness, or growth of breast tissue.[8] When aromatase inhibitors such as anastrozole were used, about 15 percent of patients were affected by

low libido, and much lower percentages experienced liver dysfunction, headaches, rash, joint aches, and fatigue.[9] While none of
these side effects threaten life or limb, they may be uncomfortable
or undesirable, which is why these meds should be taken only
when clinically indicated.

No discussion of injectable male hormones would be complete without a mention of testosterone. In recent years, an explo-
sion in the number of men using testosterone supplementation
has occurred. Reasons some seek testosterone supplementation
include replacing low levels of naturally occurring testosterone,
strengthening muscle development, or improving fertility. The
most concerning reason for testosterone use is the last one: fertility improvement. Normal testosterone levels do not guarantee
adequate sperm production because testosterone levels in the
blood may differ wildly from levels in the testes.[10] In fact, it is
possible to produce sperm in the complete absence of testosterone.[11] Testosterone taken in any form other than that produced
within one's own body is the most effective way (besides perhaps
chemotherapy) for completely shutting down sperm production.
Under normal circumstances, the signaling system within the
body sends testosterone from the testicles to the brain to tell the
brain, "We are working! We are producing the sperm and testosterone you need!" Once the brain receives this testosterone signal,
it turns off FSH and LH production until testosterone levels fall; at
that point FSH and LH click back on to resume testosterone and
sperm production. When a man is taking testosterone as a medication, the brain receives constant instructions to turn off FSH
and LH production. This leads to the shutdown of the body's own
testosterone- and sperm-making factories, the testes. As a result,
the semen analysis shows oligospermia or azoospermia. Sperm
take approximately three months to be created. Reversing the
effects of testosterone may take much longer, even up to a year,
especially in men who have taken testosterone for many years.
Men who have had testicular atrophy (shrinkage of the testicles to
the point where they no longer function) as a result of long-term

testosterone use may never resume sperm production. That said, higher testosterone levels in men receiving treatment (hCG, clomiphene, or anastrozole) increase the potential for obtaining sperm either in the ejaculate or surgically.[12]

Now, back to our regularly scheduled program. During unassisted conception, the sperm has a long journey to find the egg. The sperm must travel through the cervix, the uterus, and the fallopian tube. It then finds the egg and breaks through the egg's thick outer defenses (the zona pellucida) in order to have a chance at fertilization.

Conventional insemination during IVF is a bit easier for the sperm. During conventional insemination, the sperm and the egg are placed into the same petri dish and then left to their own devices. Both egg and sperm are in the same place at the correct time, so there's a much higher likelihood of fertilization.

The other way IVF fertilization occurs is with ICSI. During ICSI, the embryologist directly introduces the sperm into the egg's cytoplasm. Using a high-powered microscope, the embryologist uses micro tools to gently pick up the sperm and puncture the zona pellucida, dropping the sperm off in the center of the egg. ICSI is most commonly used when the male has a low sperm count, few moving sperm, or sperm with an abnormal appearance. It allows the embryologist to cherry-pick the sperm that wins both the beauty contest (morphology — the sperm has a normal appearance) and the talent competition (motility — the sperm has good movement). However, rescue ICSI done 18 hours after conventional insemination fails is rarely successful. ICSI is especially useful when sperm extraction is required to get adequate amounts of sperm. In these cases, the embryologists do not have the millions of potential sperm to choose from that are typical with an ejaculated sample. In challenging cases, perhaps only a dozen sperm are present.

ICSI allows us to maximize every single available sperm. Impaired sperm function, where numbers are present but the sperm's ability to enter the egg is faulty, is also a good indication for ICSI. Directly introducing the sperm to the egg does not guarantee fertilization or that the fertilized egg will develop into a blastocyst. Still, it does alleviate concerns about the sperm's ability to break into the egg and start the process.

Once the sperm and egg have been brought together, they are left overnight in the proper conditions, with the hope that fertilization will occur.

TWO, FOUR, SIX, EIGHT: WHICH CELLS DO WE APPRECIATE?

The next morning, the petri dishes are examined to see how well "date night" went. We expect to see attrition here, too, in that not all eggs that are exposed to sperm will successfully fertilize and continue normal development. At this status check, some eggs will have degenerated or not fertilized properly. That's *normal.*

At this point, what's in the petri dishes are not truly embryos, because even when the sperm has penetrated the egg, the genetic material from the egg and the genetic material from the sperm have not yet fully combined. When an egg contains two sets of genetic material sitting next to each other but the two sets have yet to fully integrate, this stage is called 2PN (there are two pronuclei — sets of genetic material).

After this check, the dishes are returned to the incubator. Visual inspection alone is now insufficient to determine whether an embryo should be discarded. The embryo is a three-dimensional object, and any given view under a microscope shows only two dimensions. That makes it slightly more likely that the embryologist may not be able to fully identify all the cells that are 2PN. That's why we let the embryos hang out in their dish until they've had plenty of time to declare themselves as sufficiently developed.

The next thing that will happen, usually unseen in a working embryology lab, is that the packaging surrounding the two sets of genetic material sitting in the egg (one set from the egg, another from the sperm) dissolves, and the chromosomes will begin to merge and combine. This swapping brings about genetic diversity and explains why siblings from the same parents look different. Once chromosomes combine, the fertilized egg begins to divide, resulting in multiple distinct cells emerging within the original egg's border. Over just two or three days, that single fertilized egg divides into two cells, then four cells, then eight cells, then sixteen cells, and so on.

At the point at which multiple distinct cells exist in the embryo, we consider that a cleavage-stage embryo. This occurs about three days after egg retrieval. Several years ago, the standard of care was to biopsy embryos at this point for genetic testing and usually transfer cleavage-stage embryos into the patient's uterus. Back then, usually more than one embryo was transferred at this stage (rather than the single embryo transfers done currently), primarily because the embryos were at an earlier time in development and were less assured of success. Once cell culture improved enough to support more mature embryo development, the standard of care quickly changed to growing blastocysts, which ushered in an era where fewer embryos could be transferred but with higher chances of success and an improved safety profile.

BLASTOCYST GROWTH AND EMBRYO BIOPSY: IT WON'T HURT A BIT!

At the very beginning of embryo formation, every cell is considered totipotent — that is, each cell can develop into any part of the body, from eyeballs to toes. As development progresses, that potential narrows. The first distinct point of narrowing occurs as the cells separate themselves into the trophectoderm (future placenta) and the inner cell mass (future baby).

Before this point, most labs leave the embryos alone except for the occasional quick change of growth media. Embryos are persnickety about their environment, and disturbing them even for a quick peek does not do them any favors. However, the embryos are closely examined starting on day 5 after fertilization. At this point, their trophectoderm and inner cell mass are evaluated. Embryologists typically look for the number of cells in the trophectoderm, the size of the inner cell mass, the amount of cell fragments in the embryo, and any dark spots indicating dead cells. They examine

Blastocyst

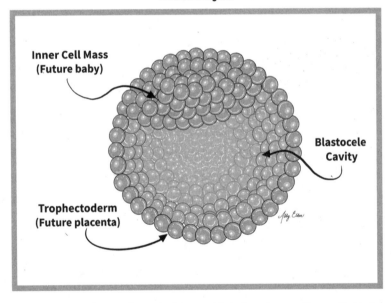

A blastocyst is a day 5 embryo. At this stage there is an inner cell mass that is the future baby. The trophectoderm cells on the outside, surrounding the inner cell mass, are the future placental cells. If genetic testing is done, cells from this area are biopsied. The inner portion of the blastocyst is filled with fluid and known as the blastocele cavity.

the embryos on days 5 and 6, and occasionally through day 7, to capture every embryo at its best for biopsy and freezing.

It is extremely common — and *expected* — to have far fewer embryos for biopsy and freezing in comparison to the number of oocytes you started with on the day of retrieval. Many patients feel shocked and even traumatized when their twelve eggs yield only two good embryos. They wonder what went wrong. Truthfully, nothing is wrong. Human reproduction is terribly inefficient. Think of it as a biological funnel effect, where you start out with many but end up with only a few. Consider this: Females start life with 1–2 million eggs, and each ejaculation of sperm contains over 40 million sperm. But on average today, a woman has only two live births over her lifetime — a good example of this inefficiency. The vast majority of naturally occurring fertilized eggs will fail before a woman even misses a period or recognizes a pregnancy. In the lab, we track every developmental step, and so the failure of an egg may feel like more of a loss because you know the numbers at every point. In reality, growth in the lab allows us to watch natural selection in progress, painful as that may be. While it's agonizing to watch numbers decrease in the lab, most people prefer to have the decline occur in the lab rather than after embryo transfer.

We will say it again because this is so important and causes so much distress when unexpected: *The number of embryos will be significantly smaller than the number of eggs retrieved. This is normal. This is expected.* Take a deep breath, and let's keep going.

Another factor that varies wildly between labs is grading. Each embryo receives a grade to help stratify its position in the lineup for future transfer. Grading assigns a number from 1 to 6 based on the development and expansion of a blastocyst. Next comes an A-B-C or G-F-P (good, fair, poor) grade for the inner cell mass, and another for the trophectoderm. As with many things in life, size matters. A fragile and puny-looking inner cell mass does not inspire confidence, nor does a scant number of trophectoderm cells, and these earn lower grades. Officially, this process is somewhat uniform. But in reality, that's far from the case, especially when comparing labs. Grading for embryos works like grading attractiveness: It's highly subjective and depends on the person doing the looking.

Once a blastocyst demonstrates proper development and an appropriate grade, a biopsy occurs if the patient has opted for advanced genetic testing. Embryo biopsy is a precise process. The embryologist makes a hole in the embryo's zona pellucida (outer layer). The hole is placed directly opposite the inner cell mass, to avoid damaging it. Approximately four to six trophectoderm cells are removed (the number can vary slightly) and sent for evaluation. Most genetic testing occurs at outside labs, because the equipment, technology, and personnel needed for genetic testing differ from what's in an embryology lab. Chapter 11 dives into the intricacies of preimplantation genetic testing.

Following the biopsy, the lab immediately cryopreserves the embryo. Two types of embryo freezing processes exist: slow freeze and vitrification. Slow freeze is the original, classic method of preserving embryos. The temperature of the embryo is gradually decreased until it is frozen. This process rarely occurs in the United States anymore and is no longer considered the standard of care. More commonly today, embryologists freeze embryos using vitrification. In vitrification, the embryo is dehydrated and then cryopreserved by rapidly decreasing the embryo temperature, completing the process within a few minutes. This provides advantages by decreasing the time it takes to freeze the embryo and preventing ice crystal formation within the blastocyst. Ice crystals disrupt the internal cellular architecture of the embryo and have destructive potential. Most labs prefer vitrification to better support and preserve the embryo's potential and integrity at a future thaw.

Embryos vitrify and remain in canes — very thin straws — that sit in storage tanks until needed. Usually, a single embryo is frozen in each cane and thawed individually on the day of transfer. Storage tanks contain liquid nitrogen to maintain the appropriate temperature. Every cane is meticulously labeled with name, date, and embryo number. Each tank is monitored and maintained carefully with manual and electronic procedures, with much redundancy. Most labs have an elaborate backup system — when an alarm is triggered, embryologists can check on the equipment quickly, even in the middle of the night. Many embryos that are not immediately needed, such as after a successful transfer, are transported to specific long-term storage facilities that house only eggs, sperm, and embryos, which is frequently a more cost-effective option for the patient. When transfer time comes, the embryo will be carefully transported back to the active lab in special cryo containers from the storage site.

So, there you have it: how the numbers work in the embryology lab. Many follicles on ultrasound are winnowed down to a few really good embryos for transfer. This is true even for the best egg donors and patients without ovarian reserve concerns. This process helps patients avoid eggs or embryos that were never destined to continue growing, and it helps embryologists select the best candidates for testing and eventual transfer. It just takes one.

. . . .

CHAPTER 11

Preimplantation Genetic Testing: 46 Chromosomes Are Just What You Need

As we've mentioned before, a woman is born with all the eggs she will ever have — about 1 to 2 million. But by puberty, her number of eggs has already dropped to 400,000. Even more surprising is that at least half of the eggs that are released are genetically abnormal. Given these statistics, it seems extraordinary that so many women get pregnant without even trying — and give birth to a healthy baby. For a great many women, however, the process of having a child can be much more challenging. We want to change the odds in your favor by helping you learn more about genetic testing of embryos.

In the last chapter, you learned about embryo development in the IVF lab. In this chapter, we will discuss the development and growth of your eggs throughout your reproductive lifespan. We will look at the way your partner's sperm enters the egg and the genetic dance that must take place to result in a healthy embryo. The heart of the chapter discusses preimplantation genetic testing: the types of genetic tests available for your embryo, which ultimately can increase your chances of a positive outcome — a healthy child. With this information, you will be able to make a more informed decision about what testing is right for you. You'll also have a better understanding of the results you receive — both what they tell you and what they do not tell you.

The chances of a successful IVF cycle dramatically improve when the best embryo is chosen. If an embryo is produced from an egg with the wrong number of chromosomes, for example, most often a miscarriage occurs; occasionally a child is born with a genetic abnormality. Here, we discuss ways that genetic testing can increase your chance of getting pregnant, decrease your chance of miscarriage, and improve the probability of having a healthy baby.

GENETIC TERMS TO KNOW

Below we explain the genetic lingo you may hear. The good news is you don't need a science degree to understand it. In case you didn't pay attention in biology class, let's start with a little genetics review. Here are a few terms that may sound familiar:

- *Chromosome.* A long string of your genetic blueprint (DNA) coiled together. Our chromosomes come in 23 pairs and are present in every cell. One set comes from the egg and the other from the sperm. The chromosome pairs are numbered 1 through 23. Pair 23 are the sex chromosomes — the pair that determines whether your baby is male or female. Two X chromosomes make a female; one X and one Y make a male. Your mom always gives you an X chromosome, but your dad can give you either an X or a Y. In other words, his sperm determines if you are a genetic male or female.

- *Gene.* A small piece of a chromosome that, taken together with all the other genes, plays a major role in determining all the characteristics that make up the person you are right now: your looks, your intelligence, and your athletic ability or lack of it, just to name a few. It can also code for inherited diseases you may carry. Genes are attached next to each other in one long string, like links in a chain.

- *Aneuploidy.* A situation that occurs when your cell has too few or too many chromosomes.

- *Balanced reciprocal translocation.* A problem that arises during the initial cell division in an embryo when DNA chains from two separate chromosomes break. In trying to fix the damage, the cell switches the DNA chains, reattaching each piece to the wrong chromosome. The result is a full set of chromosomes with the correct amount of DNA but arranged incorrectly.

- *Unbalanced translocation.* When eggs or sperm are created during cell division in a person who experienced a balanced translocation as an embryo, the separation results in an abnormal quantity of DNA at least half of the time. The cell wants to evenly divide chromosomes, but because the chromosomes are not mirror images, the chromosomes do not divide correctly, resulting in an unequal amount of DNA in each cell: some egg or sperm cells get too much DNA, and others get too little. When a pregnancy results, the embryo is chromosomally unbalanced. A baby conceived with the wrong amount of DNA usually cannot survive, resulting in a miscarriage.

- *Monogenic trait.* A trait determined by one gene. If the trait is recessive, you inherit the trait only if you receive

Outcomes When One Partner Has a Balanced Reciprocal Translocation

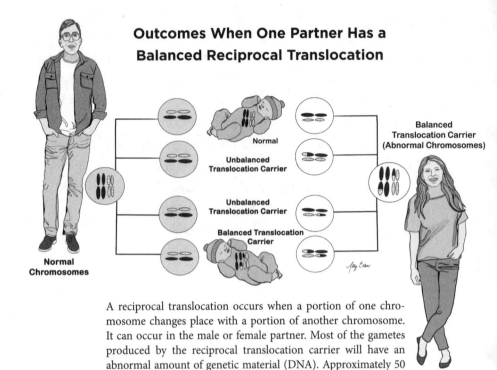

A reciprocal translocation occurs when a portion of one chromosome changes place with a portion of another chromosome. It can occur in the male or female partner. Most of the gametes produced by the reciprocal translocation carrier will have an abnormal amount of genetic material (DNA). Approximately 50 percent of children will have an unbalanced translocation with an abnormal amount of genetic material. Twenty-five percent will have a balanced translocation like the affected parent. The remaining 25 percent will have normal chromosomes.

the same version of that gene from both egg and sperm. If the trait is dominant, it takes only one copy of the altered gene for the person to show symptoms. Yet other traits are tied specifically to the X chromosome, thus affecting males and females differently due to their differing numbers of X chromosomes. Monogenic traits often come up in discussions of genetically transmitted diseases, such as cystic fibrosis. For example, if your child gets a faulty version of the gene from both the egg and the sperm, then he or she will have the disease.

- *Polygenic trait.* Some traits, such as eye color, the propensity to develop high blood pressure, and even intelligence, may be determined by multiple genes, rather than just one. At this point in our knowledge, it is usually not clear exactly how many genes interact to create a specific trait. This is an area that scientists are still deciphering for many health-related conditions.

THE REPRODUCTIVE DANCE FROM
BIRTH UNTIL MENOPAUSE

The story of our eggs and the chromosomes they contain can be a little complicated even when conception occurs naturally. In this section, we will discuss what goes on in your body from the time you are an embryo until the time you decide to make your own baby and beyond. As a cute little girl fetus growing inside your mother, you had about 6 million eggs. But the number of eggs you have steadily reduces throughout your life. As mentioned earlier, by the time you uttered your first cry as a newborn, you had about 1 to 2 million eggs. When you ovulate each month, a group of 30 to 40 eggs starts to grow, but usually only one is released. The rest die as the result of a process of programmed cell death, called apoptosis. By menopause, about 1,000 eggs are all that remain.

Once the menstrual cycle starts, the ovary releases an egg every month. Eggs often are released from alternating ovaries, but the pattern of release can be different for individual women. If two eggs happen to be released and both are fertilized, the result is fraternal twins: two separate eggs, each fertilized by a different sperm.

The egg is an amazing cell. The largest cell in the body, an egg consists of about 90 percent water. The inner core of the egg, the nucleus, is where all the genetic information is. For most of its life, the egg waits patiently for a turn to be released. During the waiting period, the nucleus contains two sets of chromosomes. However, when the sperm comes knocking, the egg kicks out half of those

Egg Cell Division

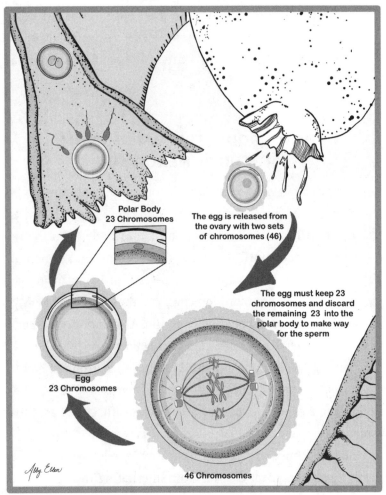

Polar Body
23 Chromosomes

The egg is released from
the ovary with two sets
of chromosomes (46)

The egg must keep 23
chromosomes and discard
the remaining 23 into the
polar body to make way
for the sperm

Egg
23 Chromosomes

46 Chromosomes

The egg has 23 pairs of chromosomes (46 total). At the time of fertilization, the egg only needs one set of chromosomes. The other set will be provided by the sperm. To discard the unnecessary set, the egg undergoes a process in which the two identical sets of chromosomes line up side-by-side and divide. This process is known as meiosis. One set of chromosomes (23 total) remains in the future egg. The other set is discarded in the polar body, which is like a trash can remaining in the outer layer of the egg. During fertilization, the egg and sperm join together and create a one-celled embryo, a zygote. The zygote has 46 chromosomes: 23 from the sperm and 23 from the egg.

chromosomes to make way for the sperm's contribution. In this process, called meiosis, the cell's spindle apparatus must pull the chromosomes apart with strands called spindle fibers.

Unfortunately, even the healthiest eggs divide incorrectly 50 percent of the time. So, if the chromosome number is incorrect, it is usually due to the egg. After all these years, the egg's genetic machinery doesn't function as efficiently as it should. If the spindle fibers break too quickly, then an unequal number of chromosomes will end up in each cell.

While your eggs are continually decreasing, the same is not true of sperm. The testes start making sperm at puberty and continue to do so, with the sperm creation process taking seventy-two days. The factory never stops. However, even though men produce sperm throughout their adult life, over time there can be changes in sperm DNA that are thought to lead to disorders like autism or schizophrenia. Age impacts reproduction in men and women, just in different ways.

When sperm enter your uterus, they swim at an Olympic pace to find the egg. Sperm can make it through the female reproductive tract in minutes! As sperm approach the egg, the tips of the sperm begin releasing enzymes. A bit of chemical warfare then takes place as the sperm collectively try to blast through the egg's shell, the zona pellucida. Around 10 million moving sperm must reach the uterus for one sperm to have a reasonable chance of cracking the egg and getting inside.

Once a single sperm breaks inside the egg, the genetic dance begins. The egg hurriedly shuts the door to all other sperm and ejects half its chromosomes (the process of meiosis). At that point the egg has 23 single chromosomes, rather than the 23 pairs (46 chromosomes total) it started out with. When fertilization occurs, the sperm adds its 23 chromosomes to produce a total of 46 in the resulting embryo.

However, if the egg kicks out too few chromosomes, keeping an extra one, the result will be an embryo with 47 chromosomes. Unfortunately, this is one time when having a spare is not a good thing! Conversely, the embryo may also get shortchanged, resulting in one fewer chromosome than necessary. An embryo with 45 chromosomes may be unable to sustain life. Many embryos with an incorrect number of chromosomes stop growing so early that a woman may not even realize she is pregnant. This is called a biochemical pregnancy.

Egg cells in women malfunction and divide incorrectly more often when the woman is over age thirty-five. Compared with the eggs of younger women, the eggs of older women begin to run out of energy, and cell division becomes less likely to result in a normal number of chromosomes. As a result, pregnancy rates are lower and miscarriage rates are higher as you age.

The easiest way to make sense of all these confusing genetic details is to think of them as books in a library. Consider each chromosome as a book in your own personal library. Let's say your mother gave you a set of 23 pink books, and your father gave you a set of 23 blue books. These two sets from your parents add up to a total of 46 books in your library. That is what happens when your mother's egg joins with your father's sperm.

If a chromosome is like a book in your library, then a gene is like a paragraph in the book. Many genetic diseases occur when both partners have the same abnormal gene and the child inherits both of them. Those types of genes are called recessive genes. If your mother and your father have the same missing paragraph in the same book, then — boom — you would have an abnormal condition, such as cystic fibrosis.

On the other hand, if you get one normal gene and one abnormal recessive gene from your parents, you would be a carrier of a condition. In that case, the disease would not affect you — unless

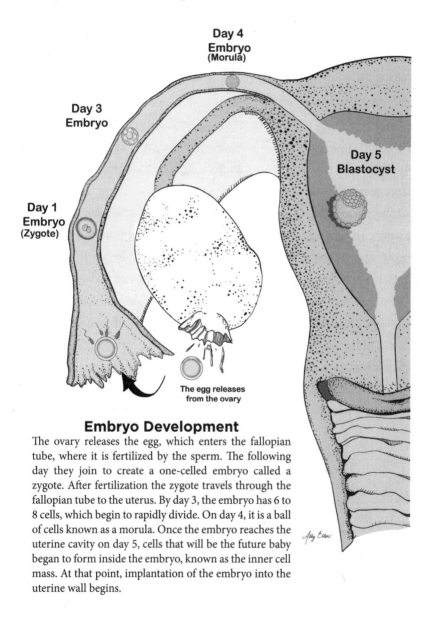

Day 4
Embryo
(Morula)

Day 3
Embryo

Day 5
Blastocyst

Day 1
Embryo
(Zygote)

The egg releases
from the ovary

Embryo Development

The ovary releases the egg, which enters the fallopian tube, where it is fertilized by the sperm. The following day they join to create a one-celled embryo called a zygote. After fertilization the zygote travels through the fallopian tube to the uterus. By day 3, the embryo has 6 to 8 cells, which begin to rapidly divide. On day 4, it is a ball of cells known as a morula. Once the embryo reaches the uterine cavity on day 5, cells that will be the future baby began to form inside the embryo, known as the inner cell mass. At that point, implantation of the embryo into the uterine wall begins.

you were tested for it, you wouldn't even realize that you carry it. Essentially, you would have one missing paragraph in the book from one parent, but a complete paragraph in the other parent's book. If you are reading this novel, you would just pick the one with the normal paragraph and ignore the other with the missing text.

As you may have realized after learning about cell division, Mother Nature does not catch every genetic change that occurs in the DNA. Even in the best of circumstances, half of your eggs have the wrong number of chromosomes. Knowing the genetic makeup of your embryos offers a significant way to improve your chances of a successful pregnancy. Therefore, genetic testing of your embryo will give you a better chance of picking the healthiest embryos and having a successful outcome.

Within twenty-four hours of fertilization, a single-celled embryo known as a zygote forms. The cilia in the fallopian tube continuously propel the developing embryo closer to the uterus. On the third day of development the embryo has six to eight cells. Day four is a day of rapid cell division, with the formation of multiple cells. There are so many rapidly growing cells it is impossible to count them all! The embryo is now called a morula. By day 5 the embryo is a blastocyst with around 150 cells. Sometimes embryos grow slower and may not get to this stage until day 6 or 7. Embryos created in the IVF lab are biopsied when they reach the blastocyst stage.

PREIMPLANTATION GENETIC TESTING

Genetic testing for embryos has evolved over the past decade, and so has the terminology. Currently, such testing is referred to as preimplantation genetic testing, or PGT. First, this testing offers a way to check your embryo for the right number of chromosomes. It can also confirm that your child does not carry a genetic abnormality that could cause significant impairment or even loss of life at an early age. There are several types of PGT, each of which can assess a different genetic scenario.

Once fertilization occurs, the embryo starts to grow as cells divide. Five days later, the embryo has a fluid-filled center and a circle of cells on the perimeter called the trophectoderm, the future placenta. Inside the fluid-filled center is a sweet little ball of cells called the inner cell mass — your future baby. The inner cell mass is attached to the future placenta in one spot.

To determine the chromosome number, a sample of cells is taken from the future placenta — approximately four to six cells. The lab evaluates the cells and a few weeks later the report shows the result for each embryo. A normal result would be 46 XX or 46 XY. Anything other than this is considered abnormal. Doctors rarely recommend the transfer of a clearly abnormal embryo.

One situation that can be confusing is a report showing that your embryo is a "mosaic embryo." This means that one or more of the biopsied cells showed an abnormal result, but the other cells were all normal. In other words, not every cell is the same — a bit like a mosaic tile pattern in your bathroom. This makes it hard to know if your baby will have normal cells, abnormal cells, or a mixture of both. Some doctors may not recommend transferring this embryo unless you undergo genetic counseling to discuss situations that could occur if your baby is born with abnormal cells. With newer genetic testing, however, we can evaluate more pieces of DNA, and fewer embryos are found to be mosaic.

Another important point about genetic testing is that it is not perfect. Remember that the biopsy samples the developing placenta and not the actual mass of cells that will become the baby. Given this fact, there is a 1 to 2 percent chance that the cells biopsied from the future placenta may not represent the genetic makeup of the cells that will form your baby. This means that if you are told the embryo is genetically normal, this information is incorrect 1 to 2 percent of the time. On the flip side, the information is correct 98 to 99 percent of the time, so it is still the best test available to evaluate your embryo's genetic material before the embryo transfer.

Types of Preimplantation Genetic Testing
Aneuploidy (PGT-A)

The most common type of genetic testing performed during an IVF cycle is PGT-A. Its purpose is to make sure your embryo has the "right" stuff. We want 46 chromosomes, no more and no less. But, at least half of the embryos tested have too few or too many chromosomes. This is the most common genetic abnormality seen with IVF patients. To use our earlier metaphor, there are 45 or 47 books in the library instead of 46. An example of a condition with 45 chromosomes would be an individual with monosomy X or Turner syndrome; what's missing in this case is one X chromosome. A condition with 47 chromosomes is trisomy 21 or Down syndrome; in this case the person has an extra chromosome number 21. Both of these conditions may be compatible with life; however, challenges are present for patients with each disorder. Common characteristics of Turner syndrome are short stature, lack of pubertal development, and infertility, while traits of Down syndrome are intellectual and physical disabilities, with varying severity.

Aneuploidy Plus (PGT-A+ or PGT-A Link)

More advanced PGT-A analysis such as PGT-A+ or PGT-A Link (the label may vary with different companies) gives you additional details about the origin of abnormal genes. This test shows if the aneuploidy is related to the egg, to the sperm, or to the embryo itself. Such results may also be useful in guiding your decision if you are considering the use of either a donor egg or sperm in the future. It can provide additional reassurance by genetically confirming that your embryo was created with your egg and your partner's sperm.

Monogenic (PGT- M)

This test looks for genetic abnormalities arising from a single abnormal gene, such as with cystic fibrosis. When the condition being tested for is recessive, an abnormal gene is an issue for your baby only if both you *and* your partner carry the same one. If both parents possess the abnormal gene, the child has a 25 percent chance of receiving the genetic abnormality from both sides and being fully affected by the condition. Going back to the book analogy, you may be missing the first two words from paragraph 5 on page 10, while your partner may be missing a complete sentence from that same paragraph. Remember that with recessive conditions, it takes two abnormalities to have an affected child, so you must look for both. When the condition being tested for is dominant, where one abnormal copy leads to symptoms, there is a 50 percent chance that the baby will be affected. X-linked conditions are even more complex: 50 percent of female children carry the affected gene but will have symptoms only if it is a dominant trait, but 50 percent of male children will be fully affected (because they have only one copy of the X chromosome, and if it is abnormal they have the disease). An example of an X-linked trait is Duchenne muscular dystrophy.

The search for the abnormal gene begins with creating what's known as a probe. A probe is a particular DNA sequence that can be used to identify an abnormal gene in the embryo. It's usually created by taking blood samples from both parents; sometimes blood samples may be needed from other family members. Using these samples, the lab creates a sequence that can be used to determine whether the problematic gene is present in the embryo. In some cases the size of the abnormal gene sequence is too large to permit the development of a probe, but this is not the most common situation; in other situations (also fairly uncommon) creation of a probe may require genetic material from affected family members who are no longer alive or otherwise unavailable.

Structural Rearrangement (PGT-SR)

This test searches for embryos with a balanced translocation (discussed earlier in this chapter) — a permanent structural change in two chromosomes that occurs during the initial cell division of an embryo when parts of two chromosomes change places, resulting in two abnormal chromosomes in every cell. Since we evaluate all embryos, we may find ones that have normal amounts of DNA and no abnormality. We may also find ones that have the abnormality with correct amounts of DNA, and ones that are unbalanced with an abnormal amount of DNA. For example, part of chromosome 5 might switch places with part of chromosome 20, a change in the chromosome structure that will repeat throughout every single cell in the body, including egg or sperm cells. This test occurs after the affected parent has been identified previously through what is known as a karyotype analysis.

This situation occurs when both parents have the right number of chromosomes, but one parent has a couple of chromosomes with the wrong DNA arrangement. The abnormality is most commonly found after a patient has experienced several miscarriages, although even in this group of patients, it is still a rare finding.

A balanced translocation is different from aneuploidy, when both parents have a normal chromosome number and structure. With aneuploidy, the fetus receives too few or too many whole or partial chromosomes. With a balanced translocation, one parent has a chromosome with an abnormal structure, but collectively a normal amount of DNA. Because one of the parental chromosomes itself is malformed, the baby may receive too much or too little DNA despite having the correct number of chromosomes.

Polygenic (PGT-P)

PGT-P is a new test that is still not available in many IVF centers. It is designed for couples who may have a strong family history of medical conditions caused by a combination of multiple genes. Such conditions include type 1 and type 2 diabetes, breast cancer, schizophrenia, melanoma, heart disease, and high blood pressure.

(The difficulty with this test is that at this point not all the genes causing these diseases have been conclusively identified.) This test is performed on embryos once PGT-A testing has confirmed they have the correct number of chromosomes. The results indicate which normal embryos may have a higher chance of having a specific condition. If you decide to test for several conditions, keep in mind that your embryo may be at high risk for one condition, such as heart disease, but at a low risk for another condition, such as schizophrenia. This additional information may make choosing which embryo to transfer more difficult and less clear-cut.

After the magic happens in the lab with PGT, you are ready for the embryo transfer procedure. Stay tuned for the most exciting part of the IVF process!

PART III

What Happens After IVF?

Preparing for the Next Chapter

CHAPTER 12

. . . .

The Limbo:
After the Retrieval but
Before Embryo Transfer

In Chapter 8 we discussed what happens on the day of egg retrieval, including what you can expect immediately after the procedure and warning signs to look out for. Now we'll discuss what happens beginning several days after egg retrieval, when the period of preparing the uterus for the embryo transfer begins.

Your hormone levels drop a few days after the egg retrieval. Because of these hormonal changes, most women start their period between five and ten days after retrieval, even if they have not been regularly getting periods on their own. When this occurs, notify your clinic that your period has started; you will get instructions on the next step. This is not an urgent phone call, and you can let them know on the next business day. The first period after retrieval is often quite heavy, which results from higher-than-average estrogen levels and a thicker endometrium than normal.

While you wait to find out how many embryos grew and the results of the PGT report, focus on you. Some patients begin birth control pills to help the ovaries quiet down and keep the lining thin poststimulation, so that you are essentially at baseline and ready to start as soon as you get the news about the PGT results. This option also assists women without monthly menses and those who want to start a frozen embryo transfer cycle as quickly as possible. Some women may have a natural menstrual cycle during this time. You may use this time to do additional testing or surgery, such as hysteroscopy, to improve the uterine lining in preparation for the frozen embryo transfer.

OVARIAN HYPERSTIMULATION SYNDROME

We've briefly mentioned ovarian hyperstimulation syndrome before — OHSS is a condition that typically starts to develop toward the end of stimulation or shortly after retrieval. If you have a fresh embryo transfer, it can also happen early in pregnancy. But let's get further into the details here, since there are ways of making it less likely that you'll develop OHSS. Even if you do, early recognition and treatment can shorten its duration.

When you go through IVF stimulation and the follicles are growing, granulosa cells within the follicles multiply and release estrogen. In some women who undergo robust stimulation, estrogen levels can get quite high. Estradiol levels above 3,000 mIU/mL increase your risk of developing OHSS. The higher your estradiol level, the higher your risk. Fortunately, though, severe cases of OHSS are rare even with high estradiol levels.

In some women, elevated estradiol levels stimulate the production of a hormone called vascular endothelial growth factor (VEGF). VEGF can make your blood vessels leaky, allowing the watery part of your blood to go into places it should not. These changes can lead to fluid collecting in the lungs (pulmonary edema) and abdomen (ascites). Pulmonary edema makes breathing difficult and causes chest pain. Ascites usually causes weight gain, makes breathing more difficult, and makes your belly expand and look pregnant. It can also slow down gut motility, leading to nausea, constipation, and a lack of appetite. Displacement of fluid from your blood vessels also leads to electrolyte imbalances, especially in sodium and potassium. In severe cases, it can lead to serious neurological or cardiac complications. It also concentrates platelets, the part of your blood that allows you to form blood clots. This increases the risk of clotting in dangerous places, such as your legs or lungs. Unfortunately, once OHSS develops, all we can do is manage the symptoms and try to make you safe and more comfortable while your body heals itself.

The severity of OHSS varies from mild all the way to severe. Most women who go through an egg retrieval have multiple eggs and mild hyperstimulation, which resolves without any treatment. If you have any symptoms mentioned in the previous paragraph, or if you experience rapid weight gain after retrieval, call your clinic; most likely they will have you come in for a physical exam and ultrasound. You may have labs drawn to determine how thick your blood is, and the results will reveal any electrolyte imbalances. If your physician feels it is safe to treat you at home, you will be sent home with instructions, including measuring your weight, abdominal circumference, and urine output on a daily basis. (You won't need to pull out the kitchen measuring cups for that last one — your clinic may provide you with a measuring hat for your toilet or tell you where to get one.) You may also be placed on low-dose aspirin. Drinking electrolyte drinks during this period is recommended over water. Also, avoid caffeine and alcohol. You need to stay hydrated to fill your vessels with fluid; electrolyte drinks help the fluid stay in the vessels. The best news is that OHSS is a self-limiting illness. As your estrogen and VEGF levels fall, the shifts in body fluid will resolve, and you will start feeling much better.

Rarely, in severe cases some individuals may need to be hospitalized for closer monitoring and treatment. Inpatient care for OHSS can include IV fluids, antinausea medications, and blood tests to check your electrolytes and the concentration of your blood. Blood thinners are given to prevent dangerous clotting. If you have fluid in your lungs, you may undergo a procedure to draw that fluid out of your lung space to allow you to breathe more easily. If you have ascites, you may have a procedure to drain the fluid in your belly either vaginally (like the way your egg retrieval was done) or through your abdominal wall. Removing the fluid shortens the course of OHSS and will make you feel much better sooner.

As with most illnesses, prevention is the best medicine for OHSS. However, despite sound medical practices, sometimes ovaries respond more than expected. This can be good in the long term, since you will likely get more eggs. If you are a great responder and seem likely to develop OHSS, some preventative measures may mitigate your risk. A common technique uses leuprolide rather than hCG at the time of trigger. If hCG is used as the trigger, especially when you have high estradiol levels, it stimulates factors that encourage the development of OHSS. By contrast, leuprolide signals your body to release LH from the brain to mature your eggs, and it helps turn off some of the stimulatory hormonal messages quickly after retrieval, so estrogen levels fall more quickly. Other medications can be used in conjunction with the leuprolide trigger to minimize the risk of OHSS. These include cabergoline, GnRH antagonists such as ganirelix (Cetrotide), and letrozole.

. . . .

CHAPTER 13

It's Cold in Here: Getting Ready for Frozen Embryo Transfer

Any good teacher, doctor, or chef will tell you that preparation is the key to success in any venture. Frozen embryo transfers are no different. Everyone asks what lifestyle changes they can make before starting the transfer process. Patients ask us about which foods to eat and activities to avoid; some people even wonder whether seemingly impossible yoga poses might help make the embryo stick! Most of the answers to questions like these are pure common sense. Here is a short list of reminders for you:

- Start a prenatal vitamin, preferably one containing DHA.
- Get lab work to check your general health: blood count, thyroid, prolactin, vitamin D, glucose, and vaccination status.

- If you have a chronic medical condition, follow up with your specialist or primary care doc to ensure it is as controlled as possible.
- Cross-check your medications! Often, some time passes between your initial consultation and the embryo transfers, and during that time some of your medications may have changed as you attempt to optimize your health. Review the medications you're currently taking once more with your REI specialist to ensure that all of your meds are safe for transfer and pregnancy.

Then there is the painfully obvious advice worth restating:

- Stop drinking alcohol.
- Stop using tobacco or other nicotine products.
- Avoid other substances, including marijuana.
- Minimize caffeine.

This is a great time to revisit Chapters 4 and 5 — the principles explored in those chapters still apply.

Now that you have done everything humanly possible to prepare your body, mind, uterus, and embryos for transfer, let's get to the nitty-gritty of the actual transfer cycle.

PREPARATION

Transfer protocols generally fall into one of three classes: programmed cycles, natural cycles, or modified natural cycles (discussed below). Each of these protocols uses medications differently, as we will see.

A patient may or may not need pretreatment for a particular cycle type. For example, oral contraceptive pills frequently manipulate cycles to help the transfer occur in a certain time frame; this is particularly helpful for patients with demanding schedules and for patients at clinics that "batch" embryo transfers. OCPs do not have a negative impact leading up to a frozen embryo transfer. In other cases, OCPs may be used with leuprolide to shut down the body's hormonal signaling system to minimize cross signals and allow medications, such as estradiol, time to take effect without hormonal interference. Typically, leuprolide is given for only one to two weeks before the transfer cycle for a little extra control of hormonal signaling. Other protocols have patients with endometriosis take leuprolide for two months or more before starting the transfer cycle to completely silence the condition; this is not mandatory for everyone with endometriosis, but it is becoming more common. A few treatments exist that have been available for many years but have never fully demonstrated benefits in studies; lipid emulsions such as intralipids (which are theoretically supposed to help with implantation) are one example.

> **Batching** is grouping all procedures in a short time frame due to availability of staff, equipment, or other resources.

If pretreatment has been advised for you, once pretreatment is complete, your clinic will tell you when to do your baseline labs and ultrasound. This may coincide with the onset of your period. This first set of labs is designed to check that your hormone levels are low, indicating no premature follicular growth. The lining of the uterus should also be relatively thin at this point, as either endometrial growth has been suppressed with medicines or the past month's endometrium was just shed with your period.

If the first set of tests shows that your hormone levels are too high or your uterine lining is thicker than it should be, stopping and resetting the cycle is very common. That means waiting for the next menses or starting (or continuing) OCPs or progesterone to speed up the process. A cyst or an aberrant hormone level is the most common cause of a transfer delay. While resetting and restarting can be frustrating, it's critical to do this, as we want to create the most ideal conditions possible in order to ensure the best possible outcome. You may want to barrel forward even if things are not perfect or if it fits your schedule better, but we don't want you to look back after a failed cycle wishing you had taken those extra two weeks. A thick lining or high hormone levels are signs that the body is in control and doing its own thing. We want the body to register only the instructions *we* give during this time frame.

Programmed Cycles

Programmed cycles use medications like progesterone and estradiol to increase endometrial thickness and trigger decidualization without influence from the body.

Estrogen

Once a clear baseline ultrasound has been achieved and hormone levels are low, endometrial thickening starts. In a natural cycle, growing follicles produce estradiol to develop the endometrium into a beautiful three-layer structure. In a programmed cycle, we use estrogen to thicken the lining. We look for the Goldilocks moment here, with an endometrium that is not too thin, not too thick, but just right. This typically takes one and a half to two weeks. It may take more or less time, and that is fine. It is more important to get the timing right for your body than to do a transfer just because it's scheduled.

Decidualization refers to changes to the endometrium that open and close the window of opportunity for embryo implantation.

Estradiol comes in several forms, including pills, shots, patches, and even vaginal suppositories or rings. These are all entirely appropriate methods for estrogen administration. Each clinic will have a specific protocol for what they like to use, and this is fine, as long as it works. Some forms may work better in some people as compared to others. With estradiol pills, you may take them either orally or vaginally, depending on physician preference and your specific clinical situation. Injections give high doses of estradiol but occasionally take longer to wear off and, of course, come with the annoyance of yet another potentially avoidable injection. Patches give sustained dosing without the peaks or valleys of estradiol pills but leave a sticky residue. Most people tolerate estradiol well. The most common side effects are headaches, mood changes, and breast tenderness.

> **Estrogen** is a general term for a group of hormones that have the same base structure but with subtle differences. Estradiol, produced by follicles, is the specific estrogen that we follow most closely. (Estrone is produced by fat cells, and estriol appears primarily in pregnancy.)

Progesterone/Progestin

Progesterone truly starts the countdown to transfer. Prior to starting progesterone, timelines are flexible. Progesterone really comes into play for initiating the final preparation of the uterine lining, making it receptive to pregnancy. During a natural cycle, thecal cells in the corpus luteum produce progesterone. In a programmed cycle, you do not have a growing follicle producing progesterone, so it must come from an external source. Progestin is a lab-created version of progesterone, whereas progesterone is the naturally occurring hormone. Either can be used alone, or sometimes they are used in combination. Without progesterone, even the most beautiful embryo is unlikely to stick. Progesterone starts the decidualization process to change the uterine lining, making it hospitable for implantation. Without enough early

The **corpus luteum** is formed from the ovarian follicle after ovulation. A functional change happens that transforms it from an estrogen producer to an estrogen and progesterone producer.

progesterone, pregnancy will fail; hence the importance of progesterone during frozen embryo transfer. It can be given through pills, injections, or vaginally.

Unlike the administration of estrogen, the administration of progesterone is a controversial topic. Methods of progesterone administration can start knock-down, drag-out battles in the IVF world — everyone has an opinion and a favorite dose. A room of five REI specialists will give you at least eight opinions on progesterone support. The two most common modes of progesterone administration are intramuscular injections and vaginal applications. Oral forms of progesterone are not used in transfer protocols because most of the functional hormone is eliminated when it is digested and filtered through the liver.

Historically, progesterone in oil (PIO), delivered by injection, has been a favored choice to guarantee full saturation of the progesterone receptors and continued high levels of the hormone, but it's a pain in the butt (literally) to administer. PIO comes in various oils, including sesame, olive, and ethyl oleate. They all work well, but PIO in ethyl oleate tends to be the best tolerated, although the most expensive.

Vaginal preparations of progesterone are commercially available in the United States. They are usually used in combination with PIO in preparing the lining for frozen embryo transfer, and in this combination the outcomes are similar to PIO only. Several studies have shown that when only vaginal progesterone is given in a completely programmed cycle, success rates are lower. Crinone, the brand name of a progestin gel, comes in a plastic applicator like a tampon. The Crinone is placed in the vagina twice a day, and the progestin is absorbed through the vaginal mucosa. Crinone is

Progesterone injections are usually given intramuscularly nightly in the upper outer quadrant of the buttock. That location minimizes the possibility of hitting the sciatic nerve with the needle. While injections can technically be given in any other big muscle, the butt provides the most real estate for an injection that needs to continue for several weeks of pregnancy. (Beware — do not try to administer PIO in your thigh! You will have trouble walking the next day.)

Tips and tricks: You can numb the area for injection with ice or numbing cream before administering the medication if needed. We recommend bringing the oil to body temperature by holding the syringe in your hands prior to injecting. After injecting, massage the buttock and use heat as needed to help with the soreness. Often, two different needle sizes are given for PIO injections: a larger one to draw up the medication and a smaller one for the actual injection. Needles are measured in gauges. The smaller the gauge, the bigger the diameter of the needle. If you use the larger one for the injection, it will not cause any harm, but who wants a bigger needle than necessary? With PIO, expect lumps to form under your skin; they will eventually go away, but it takes weeks or months. If you note that an injection site is red, feels warm to the touch, or has any discharge, or you're otherwise worried about an infection, notify your physician.

generally tolerated well but sometimes is associated with a gritty discharge. That discharge isn't the progestin but the residue from the gel that held it. If this occurs, we recommend a finger sweep of the vagina in the shower every few days to prevent buildup. The other commercially available product is sold under the name Endometrin. Endometrin looks like a large, flat pill and is placed in the vagina three times a day with an applicator stick. It is also tolerated well but can produce a watery discharge. The best way to deal with this is to stay as dry as possible by changing underwear or panty liners regularly throughout the day. These vaginal preparations are safe to use if you are having intimate relations with your partner. Commonly, you will continue progestins and estrogen through eight to twelve weeks of pregnancy, until the placenta has taken over hormonal control of the fetal environment.

The **window of implantation** occurs approximately five to six days after progesterone starts. Embryos implanting outside of that window often result in unsuccessful pregnancies.

Progesterone levels need to be sufficiently high to begin the process of decidualization. Most of the time, your clinic will tell you a very specific time to take the first dose of progesterone. The reason for this is to ensure that the embryo transfer occurs solidly within the window of implantation. If progesterone levels are inadequate or started at the wrong time, the embryo's ability to implant and grow will be jeopardized.

Natural and Modified Natural Cycles

REI specialists also use natural cycle or modified natural cycle protocols to prepare for frozen embryo transfer. These methods rely on significantly less medication in preparing the uterus, but the patient must meet specific requirements to use these techniques.

A completely *natural cycle* requires a patient with regular menstrual cycles, including consistent ovulation detected by an ovulation predictor kit. This type of cycle has the potential to be truly minimalist. You notify the clinic when an OPK turns positive, and you show up for transfer several days later. In this scenario, the growing follicle provides the estrogen to thicken the lining of the uterus. The ruptured follicle produces a corpus luteum cyst that takes over progesterone production, allowing for implantation and continued growth. While this is a simplified, romantic approach to frozen embryo transfer, this level of simplicity is not often used. Considerable time, effort, and expense are used to create embryos. Relying on minimal technology to nail down the precise timing of an embryo transfer makes many patients and physicians deeply uncomfortable, as the natural process may be faulty at baseline, leading to infertility.

A *modified natural cycle* protocol often employs both medications and natural physiology to achieve pregnancy. This occurs in a variety of ways. An ultrasound will identify the absence of dominant follicles before treatment and then at least one mature follicle after five days of letrozole. This encourages follicular growth on a specific timeline. Letrozole is an oral medication often used to recruit follicles in timed intercourse or intrauterine insemination cycles. In an embryo transfer cycle, letrozole is used to decrease estrogen levels in the body. When the brain detects lower estrogen levels, it secretes FSH to stimulate ovarian follicle growth, which then stimulates the endometrium to grow and prepare for implantation. As a result, it becomes easier to predict when ovulation occurs and progesterone exposure begins. Once the mature follicle has been identified, the trigger injection, hCG, will be given to evict the egg from the follicle and initiate progesterone production within the corpus luteum. This provides far more precise timing for embryo implantation while allowing the body to be the primary source of estrogen and progesterone. In some cases, supplemental progesterone injections augment the cycle to provide even more precise timing than the trigger shot alone. This combined approach permits smaller progesterone doses because the corpus luteum also secretes progesterone.

The data is mixed as to what is the "best" transfer approach. As with any protocol, your physician will have a preference and reasons for those preferences. One protocol or another may yield better results in the hands of any given physician. So when your physician recommends a particular protocol, there is usually a reason.

Because so many of these protocols work, there is more room for flexibility to meet the needs of any patient-clinic combination. Programmed cycles often work well to optimize success rates. Clinics want to ensure they have enough embryology staff to support the number of transfers each day. They want the embryology staff to have plenty of time to get it right and not compromise an embryo transfer in any way. Alternatively, some patients do not tolerate certain meds due to a history of cancer, blood clots, or side effects. For yet other patients, we use whatever worked in their prior successful frozen embryo transfer. It comes down to the best protocol for you and your doctor.

TRANSFER DAY

The big day has arrived!

When preparing for your transfer, you sign documents specifying any preferences related to the embryo thaw. Most commonly, these desires relate to the sex of the transferred embryo and the number of embryos to be transferred.

Let's talk about the number of embryos to transfer. In the early 2010s and prior, we routinely transferred between two and five embryos to increase the odds of success. It was truly like gambling! Part of the reason for transferring so many embryos was spectacularly average technology. Pregnancy rates were in the 30–40 percent range at best, even with multiple embryos being transferred. As a result, transferring multiple embryos was the standard of care because most would never stick and become babies. But this did result in a twin and triplet rate much higher than it is today.

Nowadays, the success rates with a single embryo transfer are much higher because the technology and the ability to do advanced genetic testing are better. With transferring one chromosomally normal embryo, success rates often range from 50 to 70 percent, regardless of age. This dramatically reduces the risk of twins (the typical twin rate after transferring a single embryo is about 1.5 percent, the same as in spontaneous pregnancies) and higher-order multiples — and, even more important, it reduces the risk of all the complications of multiple pregnancies. Women pregnant with multiple gestations experience gestational diabetes, gestational hypertension, preeclampsia, and preterm birth far more commonly. These conditions increase the risk of potential injury to the children, including intellectual impairment, respiratory distress, and feeding and growing problems, among others. Multiples also increase the strain on the parents' relationship. And, as we've noted earlier, sometimes people think that having two children at once will be cheaper, but this is actually not true; studies have found that having two children sequentially is much less expensive than having two at the same time. Today, the majority of multiple pregnancies in assisted reproduction cycles originate from cycles with injectable medication and intrauterine insemination, not IVF.

On the day of transfer, the embryologist carefully warms and thaws your embryo and confirms its survival before transfer. They check that most cells within the embryo survived and also check for the resumption of growth or expansion following the thaw. A blastocyst consists of a few hundred cells at this stage. Understandably, not all survive the thawing process, but the majority will. When the majority of cells do not survive the thaw, we worry that the embryo will not be able to implant, and we consider thawing the next embryo in line. The procedure after thaw varies widely by lab. Some labs transfer as soon as possible. Other labs will wait to see the resumption of expansion before they transfer.

Embryologists look for specific changes after the thaw. The inner cell mass, your future baby, should ideally be compact. The trophectoderm, which forms the placenta, should have no debris or fragmentation. That being said, few embryos that are transferred are "perfect," and plenty of others go on to make beautiful babies. In the best-case scenario, the blastocyst is emerging from its protective layer (hatching) or has completed that process (fully hatched). If the embryo does not meet the lab's and physician's criteria for transfer and if another embryo is available, with your permission the next embryo will be thawed and prepared for transfer instead. More than 95 percent of embryos survive the thawing process. The percentage that survive and thrive *after* transfer varies greatly depending on that specific clinic's criteria, the individual patient, and the quality of their embryos.

After the clinic has confirmed embryo survival, it is time for you to drink serious amounts of water to fill your bladder. Increased fluid intake twenty-four hours beforehand ensures that even if your bladder is not full when you arrive, it will fill quickly. Having a full bladder provides two significant advantages. The first is a clear view of your uterus on abdominal ultrasound. The transferring doc can see the uterus through a full bladder more easily and accurately, allowing easier entry into the cavity. Secondarily, the full bladder may straighten the angle of your uterus, making entry into the uterus easier (though if the uterus already tilts backward, a full bladder pushes it down even further, which is a disadvantage; however, emptying a bladder is easier and faster than quickly filling it).

In the Transfer Room

Once that bladder is full and everyone is ready to go, we take you back to the transfer room. At this point, you assume the position you know so well by this stage: feet up in the stirrups and bottom scooted down to the edge of the table. Your doc places the speculum in the vagina to see the cervix and then cleans it off with soft swabs using saline, embryo media, or both. Most doctors use an abdominal ultrasound to see the uterus clearly, but vaginal ultrasound techniques also work. If the uterus cannot be clearly seen, the team assesses if the bladder needs to be more or less full to facilitate entry; sometimes, peeing for ten seconds or drinking another eight ounces of water can make a huge difference in getting a good view. If timing is an issue, sometimes a small catheter can be placed through your urethra into your bladder to backfill the bladder with warm saline water to improve visualization. This can be a little uncomfortable for a moment but is usually tolerated well.

The ideal location for embryo placement is approximately 1 cm from the fundus (the top) of the uterus. If a guide catheter is being used, it is placed first, with an ultrasound confirming the catheter's passage past the cervix's internal opening. Not every transfer requires a guide catheter, and some physicians do not use one. It does not matter which technique is used if the embryo is placed in the uterus without trauma.

The physician calls for the embryo after placing the guide or confirming that the direct placement technique works. Typically, the embryo will be removed from its warm, cozy home in the incubator once the physician confirms everything is ready. Then the catheter is placed and the embryo is gently released into the uterus. The embryo is too small to be seen on ultrasound, but it is possible to see the small amount of media fluid with a tiny air bubble around it. That fluid appears as a small white flash that floats into the uterus. After seeing the flash, the catheter comes out, and the embryologist confirms that the embryo no longer resides in the catheter. Occasionally, the embryo sticks to the catheter and will come back out with the catheter. If this happens, it isn't a big cause for concern; the doc will replace it in the uterus where it belongs. The ultrasound and speculum will be removed at this point, and we stop bothering you — for a minute, anyway. And now you can go empty your very full bladder. Don't worry, because you are not going to pee the embryo out!

Most women tolerate this procedure very well given everything they had to do to get to this point. The transfer is kind of like a glorified Pap smear (with a full bladder!). Some clinics premedicate with diazepam (Valium), NSAIDs, or extra progesterone. There are also situations in which full anesthesia may be used during a transfer.

Post-Transfer Instructions

The first question *everyone* asks is "Do I need to stay on bed rest after transfer?" Fortunately, the answer is no. This frequently makes patients uncomfortable, as they want to do everything possible to ensure success, even if that means being glued to a bed to avoid dislodging their precious embryo. A research paper showed that resting for twenty-four hours after the transfer did not produce ultimate success rates better than resting for just one hour afterward.[1] A few years later a different study looked at air bubbles in the uterus, because they behave similarly to transferred embryos. The researchers noted the position of the air bubble immediately after inserting it into the uterus, then measured its movement after the patient stood up and moved around immediately following transfer. The result showed that the air bubble stayed right where it was placed in the uterus.[2] We hope this eases your mind. It may also help to know that when you are sitting or standing, the uterus is more parallel to the floor than it is when you are lying down. Also, an immediate return to regular activity actually improves stress and anxiety. We know anxiety and depression are not beneficial to women undergoing infertility treatment, and forced inactivity rather than a quick return to normal does nothing to improve that stress.

The second question *everyone* asks is "What activities should I avoid?" In general, the answer to this question is to avoid anything you would avoid if you were pregnant, because now you are pregnant until proven otherwise. However, most clinics will add a few other things to that list, though instructions vary widely from clinic to clinic.

Frequently, limitations will be placed on what you do prior to the official pregnancy test or detection of the heartbeat on ultrasound around six weeks' gestation. The first few weeks of pregnancy are the most tenuous, and most REI specialists give a sigh of relief after the first ultrasound showing a heartbeat. While even at that point it is still early and a miscarriage may occur, miscarriage rates drop considerably after this period. Many clinics instruct patients to abstain from sex and any significant gym activity until that ultrasound. The reason has less to do with concern that those activities will jeopardize a pregnancy and more with the misplaced guilt you might feel if a loss occurs. After all, people with spontaneous pregnancies do all manner of things before realizing they are pregnant and don't suffer because of it. The last thing in the world we want is for you to think "I caused this" in the face of an early miscarriage that genuinely has nothing to do with what you did or did not do. That said, we can think of no more efficient way to ruin a couple's sex life than for them to have sex and the next day receive the news they are miscarrying.

Patients frequently want to know what to eat, what to drink, and if they should take additional supplements to improve the success rate of any given transfer. For better or worse, no specific formula always works. The best restaurants in the world do well because they master the basic techniques and execute them perfectly every single time. A well-cared-for body is the best trick we have for success. The actions that have the most effectiveness are simple and obvious. Eat healthy foods and portions. Get adequate sleep. Look after your mental health. Follow medication instructions. Ask your doc if there is something unusual about your situation. Unfortunately, simple does not mean easy. Taking good care of your body is a full-time job, but it is one well worth doing, especially as you move through the transfer process.

One of the most critical sets of instructions medication-wise relates to your hormonal medications. If you underwent a programmed embryo transfer cycle, you *must* keep taking your estrogen and progesterone. We all know it is a pain in the butt, but that progesterone serves a critical function in stabilizing the endometrium so that the embryo securely implants. Without adequate progesterone, the endometrium destabilizes and starts to shed, causing bleeding at best (and all the anxiety that comes with it) and at worst leading to a miscarriage.

Sometimes a brief course of antibiotics is started the day of your transfer, with the intent to stop any harmful bacteria from growing in the uterus if it accidentally hitches a ride on the embryo transfer catheter. Doxycycline is frequently the chosen antibiotic and is known for causing nausea, so take it with a substantial meal to avoid that side effect.

Other medications may also be prescribed to you around the time of transfer, depending on your particular situation. Blood thinners like enoxaparin or low-dose aspirin are frequently started around transfer to help with placental growth and development, prevent preeclampsia, and mitigate recurrent pregnancy loss. Some docs prescribe steroids like prednisone as well to improve the immune response. Interventions such as intralipids and intravenous immunoglobulins (IVIG) have been around for many years but have yet to be universally adopted due to questions about efficacy and safety.

Tricky Transfers and a Misbehaving Uterus

Your uterus may seem to have a mind of its own. Despite our expertise and guidance, not every uterus grows its lining in our standard time frame. Each REI specialist has a desired endometrial thickness they want to see before starting progesterone, and some uteruses do not cooperate with the instructions to achieve it. When this happens, we have a set of techniques to get what we need.

One approach centers on estrogen dosing and route. Each doc generally has a preferred estrogen protocol, whether that relies on oral, vaginal, transdermal, or injectable estrogens. When the preferred route fails to produce a thick enough lining, a common technique is giving additional estrogen doses through another route or sometimes changing the route entirely. The decision to add estrogen, versus the choice to stop and restart, depends on how many days into the cycle a patient is and what her lining and estrogen levels are when the decision is made. For example, a woman who has only a thin lining on both patches and pills may have vaginal estrogen added in if it's still relatively early in the cycle and her levels are not excessively high. If that additional dose still does not thicken the lining, the next step would likely be to stop meds, bring on a period, and restart with a new or supplemented protocol, perhaps involving injectable estrogen or having an additional evaluation with a hysteroscopy.

Alternatively, the overall approach can be switched from a programmed cycle to a natural or modified natural cycle. This requires bringing on a period and starting over, and it can be done only in patients who can grow follicles and have enough flexibility to work with uncertain dates.

If none of those methods work, each doc has our own brand of "voodoo" we use for uncooperative linings. We call them "voodoo" not because they employ any magic but because they have a reasonable scientific rationale for working but no hard data to support them as part of an everyday protocol. This can include medications such as sildenafil, vitamin E, aspirin, cabergoline, growth hormone, and hCG. It may involve endometrial biopsies for specific biomarkers, or shifting transfer time relative to the window of implantation.

Tips and Tricks: Many of these techniques and medications have been in use for years, and every now and then they have a resurgence in popularity. For some, such as aspirin, new data may show wider benefits than previously realized. In other cases, like moving the window of implantation, new data may indicate a technique is generally less helpful than initially thought. When faced with this situation, our tip would be to run through the list briefly with your physician. We don't recommend demanding a full accounting of new data — you will be there all night. Sometimes the mere act of running through the list will trigger an inspiration relevant to your specific case. This is the ultimate goal: synthesizing all the data accumulated over your prior diagnostic testing, oocyte stimulation, retrieval, prior endometrial preparation cycles, and general medical history to lead to a potential insight that will make the difference in your treatment plan.

Once the embryo goes into the uterus, it is time for everyone's favorite game: Hurry up and wait. The next ten days, while you wait to take a pregnancy test, can feel interminable. Planning distractions for yourself and activities to look forward to will help the time pass, and before you know it, you will have your answer.

CHAPTER 14

. . . .

The Golden Ticket
(It's Positive)... and the
Lost Ticket (It's Negative)

The day for your official pregnancy test has finally arrived! First, take a deep breath. That may sound simple right now while you are reading this book, but you will probably be pretty anxious when the day rolls around. That is understandable and normal. In this chapter, we will discuss what will happen with both good news and bad news. Information is power, and that's what this chapter is all about.

On the morning of your pregnancy test, have breakfast and then go to get your blood drawn. Your lab will likely have a time by which you need to have your blood drawn to get same-day results, so be aware. This pregnancy test is a quantitative hCG level, and there is not necessarily a "normal" value if you are pregnant. A positive hCG level is over 5 mIU/mL. Although you and your physician will feel more reassured if the hCG level is over 100 mIU/mL, we have all seen successful pregnancies with low hCG levels on a first pregnancy test. Not all babies play by the rule book. At the same time, your progesterone level will also be checked. Depending on your progestin supplementation regimen, your REI specialist will evaluate your progesterone level to determine whether it is adequate or if you need more progestin.

IT'S POSITIVE!

Congratulations! Another major milestone achieved. Your REI will request that you repeat hormone levels in two to three days to see how the hCG level rises. In most pregnancies, hCG will rise at least 60 percent, if not more, in forty-eight hours at this stage. Depending on your physician and the hormone levels, further blood draws may be performed.

When your physician is reassured by your rising hCG levels, your first ultrasound of the baby will be scheduled. Based on your clinical situation, it may occur when you are either five or six weeks pregnant. If you have an ultrasound during the fifth week, you may see a gestational sac, a round structure within the uterine lining surrounded by a white rim. Within that sac, you will likely see a yolk sac — another white circle — which feeds the pregnancy while the placenta develops.

The presence of a gestational sac and a yolk sac within the uterus gives reassurance that you have a normal pregnancy in the uterus. It is unlikely that you have a pregnancy in the wrong place, such as an ectopic pregnancy (in which the embryo implants in a fallopian tube). This is very rare, though not impossible, in IVF pregnancies. But know that you usually will not see a baby during a fifth-week ultrasound, which is normal. At six weeks and beyond, a fetal pole (an early embryonic structure) will appear that initially looks like a grain of rice. If it is big enough, you can even see your baby's heartbeat. Depending on size and positioning, you may be able to hear it. Very exciting! Don't get hung up on the actual heart rate during these early ultrasounds. The part of the heart that controls its rate, the sinoatrial node, does not mature until eight weeks. So early on, a heartbeat is a heartbeat and reassuring to our ears. Repeat ultrasounds are usually performed again in a few weeks to ensure that everything is progressing appropriately. If everything looks good at that repeat ultrasound, you will graduate from your fertility clinic and transfer care to your OB/GYN. Most REI specialists don't deliver babies anymore, so this transition — though difficult — is necessary. But we still love to hear about bellies and babies, so please stay in touch!

As to early pregnancy symptoms, they can be a blessing and a curse. Some, but not all, women will experience nausea during pregnancy. That nausea may occur in the morning, in the afternoon, all day, or after exposure to certain foods or smells. All of these are normal. It is also normal for nausea to randomly get better and then worse. Enjoy the good days — they aren't a sign of something bad. Breast tenderness may occur, and this too can be variable. If you have severe nausea and vomiting, cannot tolerate liquids, are light-headed, or have a decreased urine output, notify your physician immediately. You may need IV hydration and medication to break the cycle. Mild lower abdominal cramping is also very common. However, any severe or worsening pain should be reported immediately to your physician.

Bleeding in early pregnancy is also very common. If you experience any, you should report it to your REI specialist. Bleeding can be a sign of possible miscarriage, but it is often due to a subchorionic hemorrhage (a collection of blood between the placenta and uterine wall). Cramping often accompanies a subchorionic hemorrhage, as blood is a uterine irritant. A subchorionic hemorrhage can be seen on ultrasound. With time, it usually resolves, and the pregnancy progresses normally. Sometimes a small blood vessel can get nicked as the gestational sac expands. This can cause heavy bleeding that lasts a short period of time and then gradually decreases. Spotting, often brown, can go on for quite a while — even weeks.

If you have bleeding during pregnancy and your blood type is Rh negative and your partner's blood type is either unknown or Rh positive, you may be given an injection of Rh immune globulin (RhoGAM). RhoGAM is used to prevent antibodies from forming after exposure to your baby's blood, which can cause challenges in future pregnancies or if you ever need a transfusion.

Sometimes, unfortunately, a blood test result initially indicates a pregnancy, but then hormone levels do not continue to increase. This is a biochemical pregnancy, which occurs when the embryo implants but does not continue growing. Typically, with biochemical pregnancies, once you stop your medications, you will get a relatively normal, if slightly heavy, period.

Occasionally the pregnancy continues to progress until it is seen on ultrasound, but for some reason it stops growing after that. This is devastating for both you and the whole team. While we will not feel the same sharp pain as you and your partner, your doctor and the clinic staff have become invested in your success as well, and it hurts to see a patient's emotional suffering during a miscarriage. Your doctor will walk you through appropriate options when you are ready, whether that is a natural resolution, medications, or a D&C. While no one wants a miscarriage, it is reassuring to see that the embryo was able to implant and start growing, even if it did not end the way we all hoped it would. After your uterus has had enough time to clear and reset itself, and you are emotionally ready, we will start the next transfer protocol.

IT'S NEGATIVE...

This section is intended for two groups of people: those who don't have any embryos at the end of stimulation to use for transfer and those with a failed transfer. There's no way around this one: It sucks. But it does not mean the end of your fertility journey.

If you just finished a transfer cycle, you will be instructed to stop your medications. Most women will start a period shortly thereafter. This period may be heavier than normal because of the lining prep. Let your clinic know when you have started your period so they can help coordinate the next steps.

If you did not get embryos or have not been successful with an embryo transfer, we strongly recommend that you have a consultation with your REI specialist. Though many people often want that visit right away, we often recommend waiting about a week or more for that appointment. This will give you a little time to grieve, so you may have a more thorough and productive discussion with your physician. While you are waiting, write down your questions.

At this visit, your doc will often review some of your prior testing as well as go through your stimulation, trigger, embryology reports, and, if relevant, embryo transfer cycle information. The IVF process is not only therapeutic but also diagnostic. There are things we can learn through the IVF process that we would have no way of knowing otherwise.

If you did not have any embryos, your REI will discuss alterations to your personal protocol that might improve your chances of having embryos with another stimulation. Rarely will a REI specialist do the exact same protocol twice with the same patient if no embryos resulted. There are often tweaks and changes that can potentially improve egg and embryo quality or quantity. Then, together, you can decide if another IVF stimulation cycle is the right thing for you.

If you have completed an embryo transfer cycle, your physician will often cover the aforementioned issues and talk about future embryo transfer options that may improve outcomes. If you are considering another stimulation and you transferred embryos that were not PGT-A tested, your physician may encourage you to test your next set of embryos. Even if you are less than thirty-five years of age, it's likely that at least half of your blastocysts are chromosomally abnormal. Importantly, this percentage increases with age. Chromosomally abnormal embryos are the number one reason for failed implantation, so it is reasonable to take actions that minimize this risk. If you have remaining embryos that are untested, you may have the option of warming the embryos, biopsying them, and then refreezing them. There is minimal risk involved in the warming and revitrification process, but the risk is not zero. Your physician can discuss how this relates to your particular clinical circumstance.

Before an embryo transfer, as previously mentioned, most people have an evaluation of the uterine cavity. This is usually done with a saline ultrasound (aka sonohystogram, saline infusion sonogram) or a hysterosalpingogram. If you have transferred two untested embryos or one PGT-A tested embryo, it is reasonable to consider further evaluation of the uterine cavity with an outpatient surgical procedure called a hysteroscopy; see Chapter 2 for more details on this procedure.

Your REI may also discuss other commercially available tests that may improve your chances of implantation and pregnancy. These tests are often performed on a sample of the endometrium obtained in the office through a procedure called an endometrial biopsy. This biopsy may be performed at a certain time of your natural cycle or in a programmed cycle. If you have an endometrial biopsy, you will go to your clinic for the procedure. The first part of the procedure feels like a Pap smear. You lie down on the exam table with your feet in the stirrups. A speculum will be placed so your cervix can be visualized. The cervix will be cleansed with a cleaning solution or sterile water. A tiny catheter is introduced into the uterus, and a small tissue sample is obtained. You may have some cramping or discomfort. We recommend you come to the appointment with a relatively full bladder — which makes the passageway into the uterus straighter — and to take ibuprofen (if you can) about thirty to sixty minutes before the procedure. Heat helps the cramping dissipate too, just like during a normal crampy period.

Three main tests may be performed on the endometrium. The first test looks for evidence of chronic inflammation or infection. If there appears to be too much bacteria or inflammation, antibiotics such as doxycycline are often prescribed. After you finish taking the antibiotics, your physician may recommend a repeat biopsy to ensure the endometrium is healthy. Occasionally, a repeat dose of the same antibiotic or a different antibiotic may be used to improve the uterine environment.

The second test is called ReceptivaDx. ReceptivaDx identifies a chemical called BCL-6 that may be in the uterus. BCL-6 is a marker for inflammation that may decrease implantation rates and increase the risk of miscarriage. BCL-6 may be related to endometriosis, although not all people with endometriosis have BCL-6, and not all people with BCL-6 have identifiable endometriosis.

If your test results show the presence of BCL-6, your REI specialist will discuss treatment options to decrease its negative impact. Some physicians will advocate for a laparoscopy to surgically remove any endometriosis. However, many will recommend starting with effective medical therapies such as leuprolide with norethindrone (Lupron Depot), elagolix (Orilissa), or letrozole for two months before embryo transfer.

Endometrial receptivity testing is the third option. This test looks at the number of hours of progesterone exposure you have at the approximate time of embryo transfer. It may provide insight into whether your protocol provides enough progesterone for your body or if more or fewer hours of progesterone exposure may improve your chances of successful implantation. This test has significantly decreased in popularity and usefulness as more evidence-based research has been published.

Your psychological well-being is equally important when you receive the upsetting news of a negative pregnancy test. It is normal to be sad, mad, and frustrated. You have dedicated many resources, including your heart and soul, to this cycle. However, you may need help navigating the emotional ups and downs. If you need time to emotionally heal, let your REI specialist know. They will let you know how important it is (or isn't) to move to the next step quickly. Usually, taking a couple of months to regroup is completely reasonable depending on your history. We want you to be in a good frame of mind, as we know that it can have a significant impact on your pregnancy success.

PART IV

Unique Family Journeys

The Evolving Role of IVF

CHAPTER 15

. . . .

Egg-cellent Insurance:
The Science of Freezing
Your Future

Egg freezing allows for fertility preservation when a person is not ready to be pregnant now, allowing women to take matters into their own hands. Preventative egg freezing enables young women to preserve their capacity to have genetically related children later while freeing them for other current pursuits. Cryopreserving your eggs allows you to focus on your career and become more financially stable. In addition, you will have time to find a partner, if desired, and allow the relationship to develop without the pressure of the biological clock.

Several terms have been used to describe egg cryopreservation for planning purposes, but very few do it accurately. Calling it "social" egg freezing completely ignores the fact you would not choose to do this for fun on a Saturday night. "Elective" comes a little closer, in that this process rarely has the urgency of an impending medical catastrophe, but somewhat implies this is a fun choice.

"Fertility preservation" does describe the process but can be easily confused with egg freezing when someone is faced with an imminently threatening event, such as the start of cancer treatments. "Planned oocyte cryopreservation" better represents the important but not urgent need to freeze eggs. The phrase embraces what the procedure accomplishes, which is circumventing ovarian aging by limiting the impact of time on egg quality and quantity. Women are born with all the eggs they will ever get (at least with today's technology). As we age, both the quality and the quantity of eggs decrease. Planned egg freezing captures and preserves the eggs while they are ideally at their peak capacity, rendering them far more helpful in producing a pregnancy in the future.[1]

TIMING IS EVERYTHING

Ideally, egg-freezing patients are under thirty-five when they freeze their eggs. This combines higher egg quality with the potential for more eggs retrieved, maximizing the outcome of a retrieval cycle.

Frequently, older patients come in asking for egg cryopreservation. Guidelines developed by the American Society for Reproductive Medicine note egg cryopreservation's increased effectiveness at younger ages.[2] After age thirty-five, patients may want to consider switching to embryo freezing. This does not mean we cannot freeze eggs after that age. However, we must consider the limitations of older eggs. The question is whether this process remains worth the time, expense, and risk given its lower likelihood of ultimate success.

Patients under thirty-five can freeze eggs with a high likelihood of later success. The challenge for younger patients is freezing eggs at a point where you get maximum success without overkill. Fertility doctors would love their egg-freezing patients to be twenty-five because the success rates will be stellar. That said, a twenty-five-year-old still has many years in front of her to meet a partner and conceive naturally, rendering the expensive and time-consuming egg-freezing cycle moot.[3] An egg-freezing cycle costs a lot of money for a young woman in her twenties.[4] If there is still a high probability that she will conceive naturally with a partner, that time and money may be best spent elsewhere. When a woman reaches thirty-five, we observe declining odds of natural conception.[5] The goal of freezing eggs is to ensure a high probability of success in the future, but not to freeze so early as to render the effort unnecessary. In our estimation, from ages thirty-one to thirty-four is a sweet spot to freeze: early enough to avoid a decline in quality but late enough to be potentially useful.

EGG VERSUS EMBRYO FREEZING

One key factor about egg freezing that differs from a traditional IVF cycle is the point where treatment pauses. Whether a patient goes through a traditional IVF cycle or chooses egg cryopreservation, the first steps they undergo remain the same. Both egg freezing and embryo creation cycles put the patient through the same medications, ultrasounds, labs, and retrieval process.

In an egg cryopreservation cycle, the work ends immediately after the eggs are retrieved. The lab cleans them, determines their maturity, and freezes them later the same day. In an embryo creation cycle, as we have seen, the lab combines the eggs with the sperm and monitors them in culture for a week. Embryo culture is followed by a biopsy for genetic testing. Next is embryo cryopreservation, and then a transfer cycle will follow shortly after that. Someone who freezes eggs and then decides to create a pregnancy with them will ultimately go through those same steps, but it may be several years between egg retrieval and the completion of the process. The result is similar regarding the number of embryos created and their genetic status. However, it tends to take a few more cryo-preserved eggs than fresh eggs to yield an embryo.

The difference between egg freezing and embryo creation is when you know the outcome. With traditional IVF, knowing if you have good embryos within a month of retrieving the eggs is helpful. If you do not have embryos for transfer, you can immediately retrieve more eggs. In an egg preservation cycle, you will not know about embryo development until much later. At that point, it may be too late to go back and collect additional eggs.

> A patient who goes through the initial egg retrieval for cryo-preservation before age thirty-five and does not use them until years later will have a success rate in the 60 to 70 percent range. That high success rate drops to closer to 20 percent if she needs to collect a new batch of eggs at age forty.[6]

The entire point of freezing is to avoid the negative impact of time. That works only if you collect an adequate number of eggs to potentially yield sufficient embryos to achieve the desired family size. This number depends on the woman's age at the time eggs are collected. In traditional IVF, the number of eggs retrieved from a stimulation cycle depends on the number of eggs available at the beginning of that cycle. Because this number is not inherently changed by medication, we work with what we are given. Ideally, if a woman is under thirty-five, we would like twenty-four oocytes in order to have a 90 percent chance of later success. Approximately ten eggs at age thirty-four will result in a 75 percent chance of live birth. By contrast, the ideal number of eggs you need to freeze increases to twenty at age thirty-seven and to sixty-one by the time the patient reaches age forty-two.[7] As most women in their forties will get fewer than ten eggs per retrieval cycle, you can see how the math works out.[8] These statistics originate from studies using large numbers of eggs. Statistics are good predictors when we're talking about thousands of eggs, but when we're dealing with just a few individual eggs, the results may or may not live up to what the statistics suggest.

Poor egg quality is why practicality may recommend embryo freezing instead of egg freezing at older ages. If it takes on average approximately fifty eggs to get to a live birth when you are in your forties, a lot will depend on whether one good egg is retrieved in your first cycle or your tenth. With embryo creation, you get feedback quickly enough to keep retrieving more eggs if needed. In an egg-freezing cycle, you don't know when you have gotten that one good egg until you decide to fertilize and create embryos. Ultimately, egg freezing preserves the hope of future fertility, but if the eggs do not fertilize or embryos do not grow, it may not provide the future fertility intended.

GETTING YOUR DUCKS IN A ROW

An initial consultation to discuss egg freezing covers much of the same ground as any fertility consultation. We review your history of medical diagnoses, surgeries, medication, and allergies, and of course your gynecologic history. Ultimate goals like desired family size or willingness to use an egg donor in the future influence how many cycles you need to do. Someone who might want one genetically related child is very different from someone who knows they want three kids.

The amount of testing required for egg-freezing patients is more limited than that for patients getting a full infertility evaluation. We order initial bloodwork to check for general health and infections and obtain ovarian reserve testing. The predictive value of this testing varies. In the context of infertility, ovarian reserve testing is predictive of future success. In the context of trying to conceive naturally, it may or may not be relevant if you have not tried to conceive in the past. A woman with a low egg count may still spontaneously conceive without problems. Until a woman has attempted to get pregnant for six to twelve months, it's hard to know whether her low egg count or poor hormone levels will impact ultimate success.

Extended fertility testing may be offered at the time of ovarian reserve testing. Generally, this is not mandatory, but it can influence decision-making. Tubal, uterine, and genetic testing do not directly influence egg cryopreservation protocols. That said, if both tubes are found to be blocked, we know IVF will be mandatory to conceive in the future, and spontaneous conception will not be an option. Getting more eggs now will be highly beneficial later. Carrier screening for recessive genetic conditions may reveal a genetic concern. If preimplantation genetic testing is done on the embryo, it would be helpful to have more eggs available. As you can see, while full fertility testing is not required, it may influence counseling and planning.

Evaluation of the retrieved eggs in the lab remains limited. PGT for chromosome number cannot be performed on an egg. Current methods would destroy the egg, rendering the information useless. Artificial intelligence will aid in oocyte evaluation in the future, but that technology is currently in its infancy and is neither validated nor widely used. The only lab evaluation done at this point in time is visually inspecting the egg to determine maturity. Other details noted during that evaluation give little insight into the future, at least at this time.[9] The ugliest eggs can turn into beautiful babies, and the most textbook-perfect oocyte may never progress into a blastocyst, much less a human being. Assigning future value to eggs based on appearance leaves much to be desired. Still, eggs with a particularly concerning appearance may change a patient's overall approach to fertility. This may lead to more egg retrievals, creation of embryos using a sperm donor, earlier attempts to conceive, or a combination of all of the above.

LONG-TERM PLANNING:
EGG, SPERM, AND EMBRYO DISPOSITION

A full game plan includes the steps for moving on to the next stage. Consulting an attorney experienced in reproductive law to discuss your options for disposition and the best manner to document your desires for the future use of your biological material can prevent future legal disputes. While most clinic consent forms include options for long-term planning, simply checking a box may not be enough to avoid the possibility of future litigation associated with donated genetic material where the right of use is at issue. Some patients will have biological materials (eggs, sperm, or embryos) remaining after the completion of the process—say, having achieved a desired family size, or determining that, for whatever reason, using those materials is not in your life plan. In such cases, there is no further need to preserve those materials. We do recommend a healthy waiting period after a major life event before determining the fate of these cells. Immediately after a positive pregnancy test, miscarriage, birth, death, or breakup is not the time to make decisions with potential long-reaching consequences. For example, please wait at least a year, if not two, after a live birth before making a decision. Sleep deprivation,

> **Biological materials** is a term used to describe eggs, sperm, and embryos. In general, they are seen as property, and that shapes how decisions are made. State laws vary on the definition of "property" when it comes to donated eggs, sperm, and embryos, and how the biological material will be treated when legal conflicts arise. Your physician and embryologists will be familiar with any state-specific restrictions.

physical stress, and the major life upheavals that come with a new baby do not lend themselves to calm and thoughtful decisions. Ideally, you (and your partner, if applicable) will hit a stage where you naturally know your family-building is complete and you consistently feel ready to make a decision. If in doubt, take your time. The cost of paying for even a few more years of storage is well worth the peace of mind. No matter how long the decision takes, these cells are your property, and you will decide the outcome.

Once you know the time is right, consider the three options:

1. Donate to another person or couple
2. Donate to research
3. Discard

Donation to Another Person or Couple

Eggs, sperm, and embryos are precious because of the time, energy, effort, and resources that go into their cryopreservation and what they may mean for your future. They will be equally cherished by another family that cannot obtain their own for some reason. If you choose to donate your materials, a few things need to happen. First, you must decide who will receive these materials. Someone you know personally? A friend of a friend of a friend? A completely new person? An agency that facilitates the donation? Regardless of who receives these materials, you undergo a specific set of bloodwork and questionnaires that allows for that biological material to be used by someone who is not your intimate partner. This is called FDA testing and applies to anyone who donates any type of biological material, from embryos to a kidney.

Second, the legal paperwork must be clear regarding the relinquishment of all rights to the donated biological material and any child that may result from a donation, as well as regarding who has decision-making rights over the use of these eggs, sperm, or embryos. Both sides must have lawyers who are familiar with reproductive law and who can account for potential scenarios that may arise. For example, if the recipient completes their family, can they then donate any remaining embryos to another family, and can that family discard those remaining embryos? These what-if questions shape contracts and explain why working with lawyers experienced specifically in reproductive law will save many future complications. After signing these contracts, the material and all the accompanying responsibilities pass to the recipients.

Donation to Research

Some patients want their biological material to help others, but not necessarily by creating a family. In these cases, it can be donated to research and scientific advancement. Let's say a particular cause like breast cancer is near and dear to your heart, and you want to find a research group that can use your cells to help further cancer treatment. Or if your family is affected by a rare disease, you may want scientists researching that disease to get as much information as they can from material you no longer need. Or you may just want to help the next person struggling with infertility, and that means your cells will be used by embryologists further honing their technique. If you have a specific cause important to you, you will likely have to do a little legwork to help find the best place to receive a donation. If you do not have a specific cause, the best option is to talk with your local embryology team and doctors to explore your options.

Discard

Many patients prefer to simply discard their biological materials. As with everything in the embryology lab, meticulous attention is paid to ensure that only the desired eggs, sperm, or embryos are thawed and discarded. Until you tell us the desired outcome of the cells, they will sit in a cryopreservation tank, being carefully maintained and awaiting your decision.

WHEN LIFE DOES NOT GO TO PLAN

The only certainties in life are death and taxes, as the saying goes. When a patient or their partner dies before using all their frozen reproductive materials, the immediate question is "What happens to the frozen cells?" The short answer to this question is nothing. Those materials will remain in storage until it is extremely clear what should happen next. The next question is much more complex: "Who is in charge?" Much of this answer depends on what was written down before death. Some people very clearly state they want their materials to go to a surviving partner or to parents for use however the recipient sees fit. Others will clearly state they want the materials discarded and do not want anyone else to use them. The challenge arises if the decedent's wishes are not clear. At that point, the clinic will sit tight and wait for the courts to let us know who has legal ownership of those cells. Clinics often have policies in place regarding how to use materials after the death of a patient or partner, which may inform the next steps that are taken.

No matter how thorough the patient is, life sometimes just happens. Particularly with respect to embryos, which combine cells from two distinct people, the dissolution of a relationship may call into question the fate of any frozen biological materials. Most clinics require signatures from both people who contributed to the embryo, whether or not you still like each other. Ultimately, the clinic again relies on the courts to inform us who has decision-making capacity over these embryos.

ONCOFERTILITY:
WHEN CANCER FORCES OUR HAND

Occasionally life throws curveballs. Sometimes those curveballs are covered in spikes. A new cancer diagnosis is one of those particularly nasty ones. As technology and screening improve, many cancers are treated at earlier stages in younger patients. The unintended consequence of some cancer treatments is the threat to fertility posed by lifesaving surgery, chemotherapy, and radiation. For informed patients and oncologists, fertility experts can retrieve eggs or sperm prior to the onset of toxic therapies. This experience differs from the much calmer and more planned preventative egg freezing.

Oncofertility moves fast. Most fertility clinics get cancer patients in very quickly to beat the clock. While we fight biological clocks daily, cancer treatment clocks move faster. Fortunately, we move even more quickly. Between the time of initial diagnosis and the onset of treatment, fertility docs can frequently get you through at least one cycle of egg freezing. Patients go through a whirlwind to get there, but egg freezing provides opportunities for potential family growth in the future that they otherwise might miss.

Normally, during an initial consultation for egg-freezing patients who do not have cancer, we collect a history, get to know each other, and explain basic testing. We may touch briefly on treatment types and general success rates, but those discussions typically occur during the second or third consultation and will include logistic and financial information at a later point as well.

With a cancer patient, everything gets done within one visit. We plan the initial testing we need, discuss treatment plans, review risks and benefits, and give complicated instructions simultaneously. This is not the only time you will hear the information, and many staff members will help you along the way. But that does not change the overwhelming nature of combining several fertility consultations into a very short time frame.

The first aspect of this visit is getting as much information as possible about your medical history, specifically the cancer diagnosis. It is imperative that we see you before you have any medical treatment, including radiation. Even medication that is not overly toxic in the long run is toxic in the short term. Many cancers that affect young women are hormonally sensitive or target the reproductive organs. Knowing diagnostic details like hormonal receptor status or potential cancer treatment plans helps us tailor fertility treatment to your body.[10]

The other component of obtaining your medical history includes diagnostic testing. This testing tends to be abbreviated and combined compared to a traditional fertility consultation. We need the basic infectious disease labs and some general health information to plan the cycle. Usually, an AMH level will be drawn to give us an idea of ovarian reserve for dosing purposes. Often, FSH and estradiol levels will be bypassed since they rely on specific timing to be accurate. We are very good at maximizing our information and moving on to the next step. We discuss fertility preservation options once we have the initial information during that first visit. This discussion mostly revolves around egg or embryo freezing, depending on the patient's relationship status and desires.

While the majority of medications and procedures are the same regardless of whether egg freezing is done for fertility preservation in the face of cancer or for other reasons, a few differences exist. The biggest difference occurs with medications that may be used to minimize estrogen levels if a patient has a hormonally responsive cancer such as breast cancer.[11] This is usually accomplished by giving letrozole throughout the stimulation cycle. Letrozole, an aromatase inhibitor, limits the production of estradiol, thus making the cycle safer for these patients.[12] Typically, these cycles are a few days longer but are thought to have similar outcomes.[13] Another difference includes a greater likelihood of a "random start" rather than waiting for menses to start stimulation medication, as in a typical IVF cycle.[14]

Another consideration in cancer freezing cycles is how cancer treatment impacts the uterus or the safety of becoming pregnant while in cancer remission. Uterine or cervical cancer treatment that includes radiation may not impair ovarian function or the ability to obtain embryos in the future. It may decrease blood flow to the uterus and decrease the ability of the uterus to carry a pregnancy.[15] In these cases, FDA screening procedures may be performed if a gestational carrier is needed in the future. We go into greater detail about FDA testing and gestational carriers in Chapters 16 and 17.

Medical considerations before retrieval need to be evaluated in patients with non-reproductive cancers as well. Anemia frequently impacts cancer patients, requiring attention before a surgical procedure can be done. Blood clots are more frequent in cancer patients, potentially necessitating the use of blood thinners to avoid the development of blood clots during the cycle. Some cancers are associated with masses that affect heart and lung function. One example of this is Hodgkin's lymphoma. In Hodgkin's, a chest mass may develop that can quickly block off air supply during an egg retrieval. The patient may not realize they have this mass or understand its implications for health during the procedures. Communication between the infertility, cancer, and anesthesia teams is paramount to ensure appropriate precautions.[16]

Realistically, success rates for cancer patients doing egg freezing are lower than for routine freezing patients.[17] There are several reasons for this. One important reason relates to the underlying health of the individual. A body fighting cancer is stressed. The number and quality of eggs retrieved may be considerably less than in a comparable patient without cancer.[18] Second, cancer patients need treatment quickly.[19] While delaying a few weeks to get one set of eggs out is often a reasonable objective, delaying several months to do two or more retrievals is frequently not advisable. As a result, cancer patients do not have multiple attempts to bank eggs. They get one shot before moving on to the next stage of their medical journey.

Unfortunately, financial burdens associated with fertility and cancer treatments run high.[20] While insurance may cover the bulk of cancer treatments, copays and time off from work still factor into the financial calculations. Fertility diagnostic testing and treatment may not be covered either, leading to high expenses in a short time frame. Many clinics work to discount freezing fees for cancer patients. Some charities and pharmaceutical companies may also assist in covering expenses for cancer patients. Some states instituted mandates for employer-sponsored insurance to cover fertility preservation for cancer patients. This information and these resources change rapidly, and your local fertility clinic can help point you to the most relevant ones for your situation. However, none of these fully alleviate the high cost of medical treatment.

Timelines for egg-freezing treatments for cancer patients move considerably faster than for IVF in a more controlled setting. Part of the reason for avoiding this speed in infertility patients is information overload. The other reason is calculating dosing and optimizing timing for a specific patient. In cancer patients, we don't have these options, so fertility docs apply all of their training and knowledge to guide the patient's body through a successful retrieval cycle. We occasionally do egg retrievals both before and after surgery, but before chemotherapy starts, in order to maximize egg yield. We avoid egg retrieval cycles in the middle of chemotherapy due to the negative impact medications have on egg quality.[21] Similarly, we avoid an egg collection until cleared by the patient's oncologist after the last chemo or radiation treatment.

In some cases, regardless of the skill of the fertility center, there simply is not enough time to go through a full stimulation.[22] Two techniques can serve as a last resort but are not widely used or available everywhere due to questionable utility.[23] In vitro maturation involves taking unstimulated eggs out of the ovaries and maturing them in the embryology lab.[24] Oocyte tissue cryopreservation takes a piece of unstimulated ovarian tissue and freezes it to transfer it back into the patient's body following cancer treatment.[25] As technology improves and more data is obtained, these techniques and others may evolve to benefit the patients who need them most. For some patients with hormonally active cancers or cancers that predispose them to heavy bleeding, we may give leuprolide to shut down hormonal signaling between the brain and the ovaries.[26] Treatment prevents periods, which is particularly helpful for patients prone to bleeding. Theoretically, treatment minimizes blood supply to the ovaries, and lower amounts of chemotherapy agents will reach the eggs. However, the efficacy of leuprolide in fertility preservation remains unproven, especially in special populations like young patients.[27]

ADDITIONAL CONSIDERATIONS
FOR CANCER PATIENTS

Egg disposition is a delicate but essential part of the fertility preservation conversation, especially in the face of cancer. If a patient's prognosis is dire, they can choose to discard the eggs or put them in the custody of a trusted family member. Sometimes they have the option of donating their eggs to research. This topic raises profound questions about whether you want a child made from your egg to grow up in your absence. You always have the freedom to change your mind, but having your wishes documented is helpful. While no one desires to add to the laundry list of things a cancer patient should do in the midst of the battle, consulting an attorney experienced in reproductive law to discuss options for disposition and future use of donated eggs — as well as the best manner to document your desires for the future — is recommended.

———————

Mixed among the technical procedures and the philosophical questions they prompt is one of the greatest gifts we can give our patients: *hope*. Undergoing egg freezing while facing a threat like cancer allows you to see the light at the end of the tunnel after your treatments. If you are healthy, egg freezing allows you to live without the immediate pressure to start a family in undesirable circumstances. Regardless of the reason for egg freezing, the promise it provides patients and their families is significant. The reassurance and sense of peace it gives many years down the road are unmatched.

·················

CHAPTER 16

Lean on Me: Egg, Sperm, and Embryo Donors

Fertility is a team sport. It takes a village to achieve an IVF pregnancy, far beyond those contributing eggs and sperm. Occasionally, the team expands to include additional help in obtaining healthy eggs, sperm, uterus, or all three. Sperm donors, egg donors, and gestational carriers increasingly help people achieve their family dreams. In fact, it is so common we never say, "Oh, that baby looks like you!" unless we have intimate knowledge of the parties involved.[1]

DONATION IS MORE THAN GOODWILL

Reasons for gamete donation vary widely.[2] Sperm and egg donation are valuable tools for people without healthy sperm or eggs. This may be due to age, prior medical treatments such as chemotherapy, surgery that damages ovaries or testicles (for

> **Gametes** are eggs or sperm.

endometriosis or cancer), complete absence of ovarian or testicular function from birth, genetic syndromes, or simply because the couple does not have all the necessary gametes, as with the LGBTQIA+ population. Some clinics will require that the intended parents are physiologically involved in the process by providing eggs, sperm, or the uterus, but this is not a universal requirement.

> **Intended parents** are the hopeful people trying to build their family with the help of egg or sperm donors or a gestational carrier.

WHICH CAME FIRST, THE DONOR OR THE EGG? FINDING AND SELECTING EGG AND SPERM DONORS

Gamete donors come from many walks of life. Potential donors are typically in their twenties or thirties, in very good health, and with no concerning family medical history. Egg donation from an older donor is possible but typically done only when there is a need for more eggs or sperm to create a sibling or if this is a directed donor, such as a family member or friend. Most people want to donate due to a personal connection with infertility or the desire to help someone. Many have had close friends or family go through infertility and have witnessed the struggle firsthand. Some may have no plans to have children of their own, while others have their own children and the thought of someone else missing out on the joy of parenthood inspires them to action. How state law defines a gamete donor and who qualifies as a donor under the law can vary greatly.

Both egg and sperm donors receive appropriate modest compensation for the time, effort, and risk involved through the process.[3] Egg donor compensation is higher than sperm donor compensation because retrieving eggs is a lengthy process requiring weeks of medication and a surgical procedure with considerably more engagement and risk than what sperm donors encounter. Sperm donors too must commit to many months of testing and return visits, but they experience inherently less risk during their donation process.

Anyone can apply to be a gamete donor, but few pass the rigorous screening *and* complete the full donation process. Commercial sperm banks primarily acquire and store donor sperm. Several dozen large banks spread throughout the United States recruit donors. Most patients utilizing sperm donors ultimately use sperm from a bank, although a few will use sperm from a directed donor, such as a friend or family member. Intended parents can find egg donors through their clinic, an agency, or a frozen egg bank. We advise starting with your clinic. If they do not have the donor you seek, they will have connections and recommendations regarding reputable sources.

For the intended parents, donor selection involves looking through multiple electronic profiles containing health information, family history, testing, results, and photos. Although this is often online shopping at its finest, remember that these are real people. Choosing a few key characteristics of the highest importance helps streamline the selection process. Even with favorable testing results, donation cycles are complex, without guaranteed outcomes. Prior donation cycle results provide additional information regarding outcomes. For example, an experienced egg donor with postcycle information on egg maturity, embryo development, and potential deliveries provides valuable reassurance to an intended parent. That said, this is a laborious process, and there is a recommended limit to the number of cycles a donor can complete before they "retire," so proven donors are harder to find. Every cycle differs, meaning that your cycle may not be identical to a previous cycle, for better and for worse.

The ultimate number of live births from a sperm or egg donor largely depends on the total number of completed donations. Our national society, the American Society for Reproductive Medicine, sets guidelines regarding both egg and sperm donations. The purpose of these guidelines focuses on avoiding the possibility that the offspring could meet and reproduce together, increasing the next generation's risk of genetic problems. With such guidelines, it is very unlikely for a donor's gametes to concentrate in one city, state, or even country, so there is less risk for future offspring.[4]

Proven donors are gamete donors who have pregnancies originating from their donation(s).

ANONYMOUS (NONIDENTIFIED) VS. KNOWN (DIRECTED) DONATIONS

Let's talk about anonymity and disclosure, starting with terminology. "Nonidentified" describes donors previously classified as "anonymous." "Directed" refers to donations where the donor's identity is known to the intended parents.[5] In the early days of fertility treatment, intended parents rarely knew much about their donor unless it was a family member or friend. They might know limited information, such as height, hair color, or eye color, but rarely knew details regarding personality or extended health histories. Until recent years, many parents never revealed to their children or anyone else that their children were the product of a donation.

The availability of direct-to-consumer ancestry testing irrevocably changed anonymous donations. All it takes now is for the child of a donation to do genetic testing with one of these companies to be linked to an entire network of genetically related individuals, potentially including the donor or their close relatives.

Even if the donor does not directly do one of these tests, a high likelihood that at least one of their relatives has done this testing makes them potentially identifiable. Also consider the rise of artificial intelligence (AI) and the increased use of the internet in society. Currently, many clinics and gamete banks may provide more than just extensive medical histories. They may also offer voice samples, writing excerpts, and photos. A different way to identify a potential donor involves internet sleuthing. It's amazing how quickly knowing that Donor #1234 is 5′10″, has blond hair and green eyes, and was a Division I soccer star in college in the Midwest can narrow down a search. Add a few more key details like a current job or other semi-unique interests, and anonymity disappears. With AI, reverse facial recognition searches now make it possible to find individuals just from a photograph. For these reasons, the overwhelming trend includes open or known donations so that the child may access the donor's identity in the future. Parents may disclose this information at a developmentally appropriate time. Donors receive counseling at the time of donation regarding the limitations of anonymity, and intended parents should also be aware.

In light of the fact that true anonymity is no longer a reality in our connected world, disclosure to the donor-conceived child is highly encouraged.[6] Just as children who are adopted adjust well if they grow up knowing they are adopted, donor-conceived children may avoid conflicted self-identity if they know their origins.[7] If this information is received unexpectedly at a later point in life, it may be traumatic for the child or damage the trust and communication between the child and their parents regardless of age. In the adoptive world, a secure attachment with adoptive parents leads to higher satisfaction with later relationships.[8] For this reason, we recommend age-appropriate disclosure for the child to learn that their parents had help with conceiving.[9] Several resources may help with this revelation, including children's books, cartoons, and therapists and psychologists familiar with third-party reproduction. The child then grows up with that information built into the fabric of their lives, and there is no dramatic reveal that leads to dysfunctional family dynamics. Legal contracts are suggested even for nonidentified donors to address things such as disclosure of information to the donor-conceived child or the potential for future identification or contact between a donor and child.

Directed donations, where the identity of the donor is disclosed, may take a number of forms. Some programs disclose information when the child reaches the age of majority (age eighteen), while others provide this information shortly after birth. Directed donations are becoming increasingly common in the United States and likely will become the standard of care. An important side note to this is that most intended parents and donors do not have much, if any, desire to actually really get to know each other. Intended parents appreciate the donor's gift, and donors appreciate the parents' hard work in building a beautiful family. The primary reason for communication is to exchange health information for the sake of the donor-conceived person at some point in the future.[10] The relationship between the parent and the child differs significantly from the relationship between the donor and the donor-conceived person. Communication and known identities do not change those fundamental differences in any way.

A known directed donation typically occurs when the intended parents and the donor have a more established connection. This frequently means the directed donor is a friend or family member. The screening in these cases is identical to nonidentified donation, with two exceptions. The first exception concerns psychoeducational consultation. In these cases, psychoeducational consultation sessions for the intended parents must include specific discussions regarding the relationship between the intended parents and the donor and may include a session with all parties together. The entire point of this process is to build families, not break them apart. The session directly explores the relationship to confirm that no coercion or unintended consequences result from the donation. The second exception involves written legal contracts. When working with a clinic or bank, legal consents directly address decision-making authority over the fate of any given gamete sample from the beginning. The nonidentified donor has previously released any legal rights to children produced by the donated eggs or sperm. With a directed donation, the intended parents and the donor must meet with independent lawyers to negotiate the contract that confirms parental rights and decision-making capacity involving the eggs, sperm, and resulting embryos. It is clear and expected that any child resulting from donation will be fully parented and supported by the intended parents. However, questions arise if extra embryos or gametes remain following the completion of the intended parents' family. Can those extra embryos, eggs, or vials of sperm be donated to another couple? Donated to research? Discarded? Is there a time limit for when they must be used? Discussions with experienced legal teams help delineate the agreement between parties in these cases. Good fences make good neighbors, and good contracts maintain good relationships.

TESTING THE WATERS...
OR THE EGGS AND SPERM

The process for medical clearance of a donor is fairly similar no matter the type of donor, whether they are nonidentified or directed, an egg donor or sperm donor. Later in this chapter, we touch on some of the unique points of each, but for now we will start with the commonalities. Initial screening includes a full personal and family health history, a physical exam, comprehensive bloodwork, genetic carrier screening, and psychoeducational counseling. After initial screening of a basic egg count or semen analysis, donors undergo more extensive testing, including physical examination, questionnaires, and bloodwork. The primary goal of these tests is to identify any previously unknown or undisclosed medical conditions or communicable diseases.

Of course, genetic testing is a major factor in donor screening. Genetic counselors review the donor's personal and family history for any concerning patterns. Blood tests typically include chromosomes (karyotypes) and single gene carrier screening panels. Occasionally, donors need additional testing due to an intended parent's specific needs. Most often, this relates to genetic carrier screening. Carrier panels often include several hundred conditions tested simultaneously. Several companies perform this testing. While many genetic conditions on each panel match between companies, a small percentage always differ. This poses a challenge when a donor and intended parent have tests checking a different number of genes. For example, if an intended parent carries the cystic fibrosis gene, they can be confident that the donor was also tested for cystic fibrosis, as this appears on every genetic carrier screening panel. However, not every panel checks for every rare metabolic disease, and a donor may need additional testing to confirm that they do not carry a problematic gene of interest. The sperm or egg bank, agency, or clinic can reach out if additional testing is needed.

Karyotypes check for the appropriate presence and arrangement of 46 chromosomes in the donor. Anything other than a 46 XX or 46 XY increases the likelihood of abnormalities and will be declined. On the other hand, single gene carrier panels almost always show the presence of a few abnormalities. These tend to be less concerning unless the other gamete provider has a matching abnormality.

Psychoeducational counseling includes an assessment of the donor in terms of stability and abnormalities. The psychologist reviews the donor's childhood, current living situation, prior encounters with the justice and mental health systems, and emotions they anticipate during or after the donation process. The counselor checks for additional support throughout the process. They also administer psychological testing. The exact testing varies, but the overarching goal is to confirm no clear abnormalities that would disqualify a donor.

THE FDA IS FOR MORE THAN MEDS

Once a donor passes medical screening, we start collecting gametes. A very specific set of FDA guidelines governs the use of tissue donations. Sperm and egg donations are governed by the same laws that protect the organ donation process. For example, if you were going to receive a kidney transplant, the kidney donor would have undergone FDA testing in addition to the general screening process. FDA testing must occur within a very specific timeline around gamete collection and cryopreservation. Donors answer an extensive questionnaire to determine any potential risk factors. This includes obvious questions about specific infections as well as more subtle questions related to any potential exposures throughout their life, such as travel history. A physical exam done near the time of collection identifies any potential active infections that would disqualify a donor. And, of course, blood testing for infections is done as well. This testing does not go through a standard laboratory; it must go to a specific FDA-approved laboratory held to a higher standard for donors. This bloodwork is done frequently throughout the donation process to ensure not only that the donor does not have an active infection at the time of donation but also that the donor does not develop one shortly thereafter that could have been incubating at the time of donation. For nonidentified donors, samples may be quarantined for a minimum of six months before release to allow for follow-up testing of the donor.

This is an excellent time to talk about FDA eligibility and what that means. Saying that a donor is eligible or ineligible refers to whether that person can be nonidentified. Only eligible donors may be nonidentified. A donor can be considered ineligible due to certain types of treated infection in the past twelve months or simply for living in a specific "high-risk" country for a few years. The downstream implication of having an ineligible donor means that the woman carrying the pregnancy needs to sign appropriate consent forms, acknowledging she is aware of the donor's identity and reason for ineligibility. A woman may still be able to use sperm or eggs from an ineligible donor, but that donor must be directed and the cause of ineligibility revealed. This may pose challenges if the intended parent will not be the person carrying the pregnancy. Internationally, sperm and egg donation is moving toward open, known donations as the gold standard of care, so this designation may be less relevant in the years to come.

THE INTRICACIES OF
EGG DONATION DECISIONS:
FRESH VERSUS FROZEN EGGS

Donated eggs may be found through your clinic or an egg donor agency and may be available in fresh or frozen form. Not every clinic supports fresh egg programs because of the expense and maintenance requirements. Patients working with fresh eggs typically receive more eggs, and the eggs avoid undergoing any additional manipulation during the freezing process. The disadvantage is the waiting period for this to occur. Often, the egg donor must complete some or all of her medical and FDA screening in addition to the donation cycle itself. The donation cycle timing centers on her period and her schedule. Your egg donor must be able to attend all clinic appointments and procedures and take time for the recovery process. To avoid increasing her risk of complications, she is not permitted to exercise intensely or have intercourse during the month of her egg retrieval.

If your clinic does not have its own pool of potential egg donors, egg donation agencies exist to help match donors and intended parents. These agencies typically reach farther than any clinic because they recruit nationwide. The agency helps coordinate monitoring and travel for your donor because she may not live in the same city as your clinic. As a result, additional fees go to the agency for these services.

The collection process for donated eggs is technically the same as any other IVF cycle. Medication protocols and procedures are similar. Due to their young age and high follicle counts, donors typically do not need as much medication. Their egg retrievals also take longer due to the sheer number of eggs retrieved. Typically, egg donors tolerate the cycles well physically and emotionally. In the hours following egg retrieval, the eggs can be inseminated with either fresh or frozen sperm, depending on the clinical situation.

Patients working with frozen eggs already have these steps completed. After egg retrieval, eggs are divided into "lots" (usually between five and ten eggs) and become available to intended parents. This is a much more convenient method because there's little waiting involved once the donor selection has been made. Eggs often need to be shipped to your clinic, depending on where they originate. The egg bank will likely do a training session to ensure that the clinic knows how to thaw the eggs properly, because not all thawing processes are the same. Once the eggs arrive at the clinic, they are warmed, insemination occurs, and embryos develop.

The disadvantage of working with frozen eggs is the relatively small number of eggs available in each group. You can buy multiple lots simultaneously, but it increases your costs accordingly. The other disadvantage is that eggs are more technically difficult to work with than an embryo. As discussed in Chapter 15, not every egg survives the thaw. Eggs consist of a single cell, compared to an embryo consisting of 150 to 300 cells. This impacts the egg's stability. Also, eggs are earlier in the developmental process. You cannot tell whether the egg will become an embryo simply by looking at it. No testing currently exists to look at any eggs, fresh or frozen, to determine if they are good before selecting them, although new research may help.[11] AI technologies to evaluate gametes (eggs and sperm) exist but remain experimental.

The "fresh versus frozen" debate often occupies significant brain space for patients needing donor eggs. Frozen eggs help those who are on a stricter timeline (every fertility patient wants to be pregnant yesterday, but someone awaiting a hysterectomy for cancerous cells has a different sense of urgency). They also can be helpful for patients who want only one child or who have had difficulty in completing a donation with a fresh donor. Fresh donations especially help when a significant male factor (such as a severely low sperm count or poor motility) impacts the sperm and you need every possible advantage to obtain an embryo. Fresh eggs offer advantages when advanced genetic testing or a desired large family size depends on higher numbers of available embryos. Patients requiring PGT-M (a test for single gene defects) will find that a greater percentage of embryos are unusable, making a higher number of available embryos desirable.

Regardless of whether you start with fresh or frozen eggs, success rates with donated eggs tend to be quite high. The primary reason for this relates to the donor's age at the time of egg collection. That said, "high" is different from "100 percent." Even in the best-case scenarios, not every egg makes an embryo. Generally, when working with frozen eggs, having a few extra eggs is helpful.

Once the embryo is created, the fresh versus frozen status of the eggs no longer matters. Even beautiful, genetically tested embryos do not always result in a live birth. It is tempting to be lulled into complacency when using an egg donor, assuming guaranteed success, but human reproduction remains inefficient even in ideal situations.

The pitfalls of egg donation all lead back to the same thing: the possibility of no live birth. Potential reasons for no live births vary. The most frustrating part for intended parents is probably when the donor does not complete the donation for some reason. An incomplete donation rarely occurs once a donor starts medications. More often, she stops due to failing medical screening or experiencing a life change preventing donation, such as a different job, new partner, new health issue, or unexpected pregnancy. Of course, it is always possible that an egg donation cycle does not produce embryos or a live birth simply due to the inefficiency of human reproduction.

SMALL BUT IMPORTANT DETAILS
ABOUT TINY SWIMMERS

Collection and cryopreservation of samples occur after sperm donor selection and screening. A standard single semen collection yields more than 40 million moving sperm.[12] In the context of fertility treatment, we typically do not need all 40 million at one time. As a result, each sperm collection is divided into separate vials. The preparation of each vial differs based on the ultimate treatment type and may involve more extensive testing such as a SpermQT. "Washing" refers to separating the sperm from the seminal fluid. This is far more relevant with intrauterine insemination, due to the makeup of the seminal fluid; it has nothing to do with being "clean" or "dirty." However, using washed sperm may lower the risk of sexually transmitted diseases, which are carried mostly in the seminal plasma. IVF and IUI samples use washed sperm, and samples for home insemination use unwashed sperm. Vials for use with IVF and ICSI tend to have much lower sperm counts than the minimum 5–10 million sperm found in washed IUI vials. That's because when you need only a dozen good sperm, having 10 million sperm does not provide much benefit compared to having one million sperm. Such vials are usually labeled as "ART," "ICSI," or "IVF" and are usually less expensive.

CYTOMEGALOVIRUS TESTING

Cytomegalovirus (CMV) testing always pops up as a question for people choosing sperm donors due to its inclusion as a search criterion on donor websites. This type of virus causes symptoms of a common cold. Sperm testing includes CMV because, as we mentioned before, sperm donation follows the same rules as solid organ donation. When someone receives a solid organ donation, their immune system must be completely shut down. Otherwise, their body rejects that organ. In that case, getting a cold virus can be life-threatening. In the case of using a sperm donation, the person receiving the donation is perfectly healthy, and CMV therefore poses little threat.

There is a theoretical risk that CMV could get transferred through a sperm donation. Sperm donors are screened for CMV antibodies to determine whether they have previously had this infection; they're not sick at the time of collection, but a virus could be present in seminal fluid and pass to the recipient. The reason we worry about this is that a woman who has CMV during the first trimester may have a child with significant birth defects. It is a theoretical risk, but it's there, so to be thorough, we discuss it. This tends to be of more concern with insemination cycles than with IVF.

We test the recipient for CMV IgG antibodies (the antibodies that show immunity and past infection) to help patients know whether they need a CMV-negative or CMV-positive sample. If the female patient has antibodies of her own, it doesn't matter whether the donor is positive or negative because she has her own built-in protection with those antibodies. However, if she does not have antibodies, the safest recommendation is to work with a CMV-negative donor. The risk of using a CMV-positive donor in a CMV-negative woman is minimal but one that should be discussed with your doctor.

PRACTICAL MATTERS: GETTING SPERM TO THE CLINIC

Once you have identified your sperm donor of choice, the next project involves shipping the sample to your clinic. You will work directly with the cryobank to identify the sperm donor and pay for the specific vials. Your clinic will need to fill out a certain set of forms, allowing the sperm to be shipped to them for appropriate storage. This is routine for clinics. Just give them the forms, which will be quickly completed and returned to the sperm bank.

The number of vials to buy varies from patient to patient. Ultimate family goals, treatment methods, and the likelihood of success all influence the number of vials to buy. A twentysomething woman with PCOS undergoing IVF probably needs only one small vial to establish her whole family, although it is always good to have at least one backup vial. A forty-three-year-old planning intrauterine insemination will likely need a great many vials to reach her goal, given success rates for women in their forties.

When you do choose your sperm donor, hang on to your list of potential donors, as sperm samples can sell out, and it's helpful to have your original list if you need to move on to your second or third choice. Sometimes a couple will run out of sperm while attempting to expand their family. If that describes your situation, reach out to the sperm bank. They may be able to ask if the donor is willing to give additional specimens.

EMBRYO DONATION

Embryo donation has increased considerably in the past few years as awareness of its availability increases.[13] Embryo donation occurs when extra embryos remain after completing family-building. Given the unpredictable nature of human growth and development, we do not know exactly how many embryos it will take to get to the desired number of live births for a given family. In some cases, we are fortunate enough to have extra embryos after the family has grown to its desired size. Some families choose to donate these embryos to other people in need of fertility treatment.

The process of embryo donation follows the same testing principles as egg or sperm donation. The primary difference with FDA testing in embryo donation is that this testing occurs well after the embryos have been made rather than before the eggs or sperm have been retrieved. After the donors complete the risk assessment, potential recipients receive this information. The people involved complete contracts delineating ownership and decision-making capacity over the embryos. The American Society for Reproductive Medicine recommends a psychoeducational evaluation for all parties involved. If obtaining donor embryos from an embryo bank, you may need to have a home study and create a portfolio for potential donating couples to peruse. Other banks, often those within fertility clinics, may not require these steps. As with any donation, the potential exists for the donor-conceived child to identify the donor(s) later in life, and age-appropriate disclosure is recommended. From that point forward, frozen embryo transfers continue as they would for any patient.

Available selection is the major difference between egg or sperm donation versus embryo donation. With egg or sperm donation, the intended parent can select donors with specific characteristics important to the recipient. You can often get close to the characteristics most important to you. When that occurs with both the egg provider and the sperm provider, the recipient couple has a better chance of having a child that resembles them. That is never 100 percent guaranteed, because genetic variations always exist, but it is more likely when you can specify traits. Donor embryos do not provide that same selection flexibility. Rarely does a recipient have an extremely wide population of embryos from which to choose. This results in far less availability for specific selections. The characteristics of the donating couple play a large role in success as well. The age of the oocyte and sperm provider significantly impacts success rates, as do other relevant diagnoses such as endometriosis or PCOS. PGT results may or may not be available.

Depending on when the embryo was frozen, it may have been vitrified or slow-frozen. Slow freezing was the standard of care for many years before vitrification but has lower success rates. As a recipient, you do not control the choice of the originating embryology lab and so cannot take into consideration its success rates. All of this is to say that donor embryos can be very helpful in establishing your family, but choices may be more limited than when using an egg or sperm donor.

Embryo donors can be found through clinics, websites, social media, or specific embryo donation agencies. Many agencies have specific requirements surrounding potential recipients that may heavily consider marital status or other nonmedical factors. This, along with the relatively low number of embryos to adopt, makes embryo donation a bit trickier to complete than many couples anticipate. The most significant advantage of embryo donation lies in the considerably decreased cost of the process. Many states do not have specific laws addressing embryo donation. It is highly recommended that when embryo donation is a consideration (either you are someone seeking to donate remaining embryos or you are considering utilizing donated embryos to create your family) you obtain a consultation with an experienced reproductive law attorney before taking action. An experienced attorney can provide advice on the legal options that may be available to you and can prepare appropriate legal contracts for your situation.

Once we have an embryo or all the components to make an embryo (eggs and sperm), the next step is to find a happy home for the next nine months. Unfortunately, not every future parent has the ability to carry their own child, so our next chapter dives into gestational carriers.

CHAPTER 17

·················

An Oven for the Bun:
Gestational Carriers

Creating a viable embryo is a critical step in the journey to a successful pregnancy, and the home for that embryo is just as important. Unfortunately, not every parent has the capacity to carry their own child. Single males, male couples, or people assigned male at birth simply do not have the correct organs to grow a baby. For people assigned female at birth, a variety of conditions can negatively impact their ability to carry a child. Uterine anomalies may alter the shape of the uterus, rendering it inhospitable. Heart-shaped or unicornuate uteri that are only half the size of a normal uterus may lack the capacity to expand and accommodate a growing baby. For patients with uterine agenesis, the uterus never develops in the first place. Radiation given during cancer treatment may destroy the endometrial lining, and surgical removal of the uterus for any reason ends the endeavor before it begins. In some cases, illness prevents a woman from carrying the pregnancy. Severe conditions like pulmonary hypertension, aortic stenosis, or certain congenital abnormalities hold an unacceptably high risk of death for any woman who attempts pregnancy. This list touches on only a smattering of reasons for using a gestational carrier (GC).[1]

Whatever the reason, gestational carriers help families who obtain embryos but do not have the ability to carry them. These embryos may originate from the intended parents' eggs and sperm, egg or sperm donors, or embryo donors. The one unifying principle of working with a gestational carrier is that her eggs are not used in embryo creation, and she has no genetic relationship to the child she is carrying. This means IVF is the only method by which gestational carriers can be utilized.[2]

Gestational surrogacy differs from traditional surrogacy. Traditional surrogacy utilizes the egg of the woman carrying the pregnancy as well as her uterus. This opens the door for possible disputes once the child is born because the woman carrying the pregnancy has a genetic relationship with the child. It also increases the opportunity for an emotional attachment, which complicates releasing the child to its intended parents. Some states will award the carrier parental custody regardless of the original intention of the relationship. As a result, traditional surrogacy occurs in some states but is less frequently done due to potential legal implications. Many clinics decline to do traditional surrogacy, and many states prohibit it.[3] In this chapter, we refer exclusively to gestational carriers doing gestational surrogacy.

ON THE SEARCH: FINDING A GC

Many relationships between intended parent and GC are established through surrogacy agencies. Agencies help facilitate relationships by finding and vetting potential GCs, finding potential intended parents (IPs), performing a preliminary evaluation on the GC for her suitability to complete this process, and helping both sides navigate the legal and financial landscape of gestational surrogacy. Agencies also know which states to avoid because they have unfavorable laws for surrogacy, establishing parentage, or women's healthcare in general.

Independent journeys without an agency also exist. While independent journeys may be more cost-effective, they are more time-intensive for both the surrogate and the intended parents. Sometimes, logistics are handled exclusively by the intended parent; at other times, they are coordinated through nurses at the fertility clinic. This includes background checks, travel arrangements, monitoring clinic appointments, payment, record transfer, and problem-solving when the unexpected occurs. If an agency is not used, it is critical to find an attorney specializing in reproductive law to handle the legal aspects. The attorney needs to be in the state in which the carrier will deliver since laws vary from state to state.

Often, intended parents underestimate the amount of time it takes to set up appointments and the education that must occur for both parties in this process, from medical clearance to delivery. The sheer amount of information to be communicated is so voluminous and important that there's no way to do it in one or two sessions. A great many questions arise requiring input from a variety of professions. The world of third-party reproduction is relatively small, and the professionals who work with it generally know who is to be trusted. The overall process of finding and medically clearing a GC easily takes six to twelve months or more when you account for everything that must fall into line.

One of the most important steps includes finding a GC who meets all the criteria. The American Society for Reproductive Medicine lists clear criteria for consideration to begin the medical clearance process.[4] The recommended age for GCs is between twenty-one and forty-five years. Relationships and living situations must be stable. Her financial situation must be secure enough (for example, not on any government assistance) to avoid any possibility of coercion or exploitation. In certain states participation as a GC may be limited by current marital status and the willingness of a spouse to participate in the process. One of the most important considerations is her prior pregnancy history. The GC must have had at least one full-term live birth and be in good health both physically and mentally. Another very important consideration for selecting a GC is her psychological capacity to carry the pregnancy and then hand the child to the intended parents immediately afterward. Some women who have not had children may be willing to be a surrogate, especially for a friend or family member. But with no idea how their bodies will handle pregnancy or how they may emotionally feel after carrying a pregnancy, it is generally not recommended. On the other hand, more is not always better. A GC who has had multiple cesareans with previous deliveries may be excluded because she could be at higher risk for uterine rupture, a dangerous situation for both GC and baby. Similarly, a woman who has had multiple deliveries is at a higher risk for life-threatening bleeding after delivery. Definitely include your clinical team as you select a GC to help vet these concerns.

Interestingly, the location of the GC's home as related to either the clinic or the intended parents is not usually an important consideration. While having them in the same place is convenient and potentially cost-saving, it rarely occurs. The intended parents, clinic, GC, and agency often are based in separate states or even countries. Fortunately, telemedicine makes fluid care possible.

A far more important criterion than location is whether the GC's personality and approach to surrogacy align with that of the IP(s). A surrogate who wants a close, ongoing, almost familial relationship with the IPs and their growing family is very different from one who views this as more of a transactional relationship. Neither is better nor worse, but a mismatch in this respect between IPs and GC will inevitably result in hurt feelings and conflict.

Pregnancy can be a very emotional time, and aligned perspectives will decrease the chance of unexpected conflict.

DETAILS, DETAILS, DETAILS:
THE MEDICAL CLEARANCE

After a GC candidate is identified, her medical records are reviewed. The medical record review includes obtaining information from obstetricians' offices and hospitals involved with her previous deliveries. We cross-check these records because even the most medically savvy patients may not have understood or known everything that was being monitored during their pregnancy care and delivery. Obtaining these records can be daunting, particularly with the time required to get them in their entirety from all relevant places.

A medical screening visit is scheduled once the initial medical record review and approval are complete. This visit often takes a couple of hours in the clinic. During this visit, all components of the potential GC's medical history are reviewed. Even conditions seemingly unrelated to pregnancy are important because of their potential impact on the pregnancy. We get vital signs and perform a physical exam. A saline ultrasound or hysteroscopy evaluates the uterine lining for polyps, fibroids, or other abnormalities that can interfere with pregnancy. These conditions are often silent. While they may not impact the GC's overall health, polyps and fibroids tend to bleed and may interfere with healthy implantation, so we want to remove them to create a perfect nursery for your embryo to call home for nine months. If the medical screening visit occurs after her period but before ovulation, the lining should be thick with a distinctive three-layer appearance. If it does not have that appearance, it does not mean she cannot be a GC, but we may need further evaluation before giving final medical approval.

An essential component of the medical clearance visit includes discussions of risks and how the process works. Many surrogates will have an idea of possible risks before setting foot in the clinic — and, frankly, they should. However, this information is frequently obtained from the internet, agencies, or other surrogates rather than medical professionals. The physician needs to walk through the process with the potential GC and answer her questions while making the potential risks of this process crystal clear. Clinics and agencies intentionally choose GCs for their good health and uncomplicated pregnancies. That said, every pregnancy is different. One challenging aspect of obstetrics is that an otherwise completely uneventful pregnancy with no risk factors may change in the span of two minutes or less when a baby or GC is in distress, so thorough counseling in advance is paramount.

This counseling typically has three parts. The first part describes what happens, including the timeline, medications, and procedures. The second part reviews the risks of those medications, procedures, and the pregnancy itself. Many people fail to realize the complexity and risk inherent in a normal pregnancy. While REI specialists do not want to frighten a potential GC unnecessarily, we do want to ensure she knows the risks, even if her own pregnancies were super easy. Pregnancy is the most dangerous thing most women will ever experience. Risks such as miscarriages, procedures like a D&C or C-section, medication and advanced monitoring, and even death should be included in this discussion. Obviously, if we think someone is more likely to have any of those complications, we say "no, thank you" to her application. But the tricky part about obstetrics is that those complications can occur even in the healthiest young women without warning. The third part of counseling addresses FDA testing results. This part incorporates the discussion of eligibility or ineligibility we mentioned in the prior section about donors. Rarely does this discussion change the course of treatment. If one or both parents have a significant medical condition that potentially impacts the GC's health (such as HIV or other infections), the GC must know this from the beginning of the arrangement. The medical visit serves to answer any lingering questions.

After completing the medical screening visit, we await laboratory results. These results look at general health conditions such as diabetes, thyroid function, infections, and anemia. During this time, the GC also undergoes psychiatric evaluation to ensure she is a good candidate for carrying another family's child. We give final medical clearance after reviewing all results and addressing any issues.

LEGAL CLEARANCE: GOOD CONTRACTS PRESERVE GOOD RELATIONSHIPS

After medical clearance is completed, legal clearance begins. We recommend waiting to start legal clearance until medical clearance occurs, to avoid unnecessary expenses if medical clearance is denied. This process occurs between the GC, the IPs, and lawyers for both sides. Each party needs its own lawyer; the GC and IPs cannot have the same attorney. We cannot stress enough how significantly having a lawyer specifically experienced in third-party reproduction impacts this process. While many types of lawyers can draw up a contract, not all of them have the experience to know what type of problems may arise or draft contracts to provide for these contingencies. This is not the time to use a contract template found on the internet. Even if the surrogate and IPs have a preexisting relationship (*especially* if they have a preexisting relationship!), good contracts and arrangements ahead of time will help ensure those relationships are preserved.

One example of the situations an experienced lawyer can help you deal with is a GC traveling during pregnancy. Even if a contract clearly states that the intended parents will retain all parental rights after delivery, not every state upholds that agreement. Certain states favor the GC if she asserts parental rights at the time of delivery, even if she has no genetic relationship with the child. A thorough contract specifically delineates where and when travel is permitted to avoid these issues.

A thorough contract also clearly details a reimbursement timeline for the process. No one wants to feel either cheated or slighted during this journey. Typically, reaching specific milestones results in a payment.

Part of this clearance process confirms financial arrangements and timeline. Financial considerations include reimbursement for the surrogate and additional provisions for potential events. It is not enough to say that the GC will receive the agreed-upon fee upon delivery of the child. While it would be fantastic for the process to work perfectly every time, negative pregnancy tests, miscarriages, and pregnancy complications can occur. These situations impact the surrogate's life and health, and their reimbursement varies accordingly. Even an uncomplicated cesarean delivery impacts the surrogate very differently than an uncomplicated vaginal delivery. The contract also includes expenses such as maternity clothes and childcare as well as medical and life insurance for the surrogate.

A GC with her own health insurance policy may not be able to access it for surrogacy-related care. Special policies exist specifically for surrogates. Similar considerations exist for the newborn. The child will not be covered under the surrogate's insurance, so ensuring there is a plan to cover the child's medical expenses is critical for both good outcomes and avoiding unpleasant financial surprises. Some hospitals adept at surrogate cases will have cash pricing plans in place for delivery, but not necessarily for unexpected complications with the baby requiring more than the standard newborn care. In the event of a prolonged NICU stay, these expenses can exceed hundreds of thousands of dollars. Planning for such contingencies helps avoid financial and medical disasters.

The funds to provide for this care are typically set aside in advance. The surrogate needs assurance that she will not be stuck with hospital bills for these expenses and that the intended parents have the ability to compensate her for the risk she is undertaking. Parents require assurance that the GC will not just take the money and run without fulfilling her end of the bargain. To address these concerns, funds are often held by a third party. Occasionally, this is done by the surrogacy agency. A safer approach from a legal stand-point is for the funds to be held in a reputable escrow account until they are disbursed. This assures everyone involved that the available money is distributed only after the appropriate completion of a segment of the journey.

Within the contract, things such as nutrition, exercise, and perhaps work or hobbies may be addressed. Some of the principles around medical care will also be included, particularly regarding a possible elective C-section or a vaginal birth after a C-section. The location of delivery may also be included in this contract. Late in the third trimester is not the time to find out that a GC wants a home birth while the intended parents want a hospital birth with an adjacent NICU.

Every GC contract discusses the essential topic of termination of pregnancy. Although access to termination may not be available in every jurisdiction, in gestational surrogacy many of the relation-ships cross state lines, and it is still important to have this discus-sion between IPs and the GC. Even with the best possible advanced genetic screening and testing, serious medical conditions may arise for the GC or the baby. Though many IPs will have PGT per-formed on their embryos, no testing is perfect. Additionally, many birth defects that can be diagnosed during midpregnancy are not related to the genetics of the parents. For example, significant heart defects cannot be picked up at the embryonic stage because the heart does not yet exist, but their presence wildly impacts the outcome of the pregnancy. From a different angle, severe preeclampsia early in pregnancy, before the child can survive outside the womb, may threaten the GC's life. The importance of thoroughly discussing these possibilities before taking the first medication cannot be stressed enough. No one can force a GC to terminate a pregnancy, but she also will not have responsibility for an exceptionally medically complex child after delivery. This delicate balance must be approached with frank discussion and grace to ensure a good match between the GC and the intended parents.

Another essential consideration is legal parentage. The process of obtaining birth certificates containing the parents' names differs by county, state, and country. In some areas, parents may obtain a pre-birth order that allows for intended parents to be confirmed as the legal parents of the child and included as the child's parents on the birth certificate at the time of birth. In other areas, the GC will need to be listed on the child's birth certificate and then removed and replaced by an intended parent after birth, and this process may take several weeks. In any case, parents typically cannot obtain passports or travel internationally with their newborn until they have received a formal birth certificate. Domestic travel may also be impacted if a birth certificate is not available in the names of the intended parents. Travel and parentage issues are compounded when multiple countries are involved. If the IPs and the surrogate live in different countries, it is vital to consult with attorneys in both countries as early as possible in the gestational surrogacy process to ensure the IPs are aware of all the legal considerations. International laws and sentiments surrounding assisted reproduction and third-party reproduction vary substantially and impact who may use the services and who may not. In any case, anticipate spending several weeks (or months, in the case of international parents) in the location of the birth to allow time for documentation to be completed and official.

Unfortunately, not every GC journey goes smoothly. Match breaks between IPs and GCs occur due to a variety of factors. Sometimes ideological differences, financial differences, or poor timing result in having to find a new GC, who then has to be screened. Occasionally, despite everyone's best efforts, the GC's endometrium does not thin out or thicken up appropriately. In those cases, alternative protocols are attempted, but if it just does not work, a match break may occur.

Medical complications may prevent a GC from continuing her journey. A newly diagnosed illness or unexpected medical event may completely disqualify her from continuing despite previously passing all her screenings. First and foremost, we must return the GC to her own family in good condition. Given the elective nature of this process, if a GC is at risk, it is much better to stop and restart with someone new despite the time and energy it takes. Clinics take their roles as medical professionals very seriously. We hate breaking IP-GC matches but have unique and extensive experience with pregnancies to guide decision-making. While a match break is disappointing, a phone call announcing the loss of life is far worse. Please trust our good intentions and 360-degree view.

EXECUTING THE PLAN:
LET'S GET PREGNANT!

Now that an immense amount of work, time, and money has been spent finding a suitable GC, it is time to get her pregnant!

GC cycles work similarly to any other frozen embryo transfer. Medication protocols vary from clinic to clinic but tend to be standard. However, one unique factor about GC cycles is that monitoring usually occurs close to her home rather than at the clinic housing the embryos. It takes an extra layer of clinic staff to send orders to an outside location and chase down those results. Not only do the clinic staff need to communicate instructions to the GC, but they also need to update the IP(s) and agency. We have found it incredibly helpful over the years to have GCs request that a photograph of their lining be taken during their ultrasound. This image can then be sent quickly to determine the next steps. Labs are also needed, but we can figure out a lot from one good picture of the lining.

GCs often use a suppressive medication such as leuprolide and/or birth control pills leading into their transfer cycles to help nail down the timing. When they get their period, they go to their monitoring clinic for baseline labs and ultrasounds to ensure the uterus and ovaries are quiet. At that point, we typically start estrogen. About a week or two later, labs determine hormone levels, and ultrasounds assess endometrial thickness. Once the lining is perfect, we start progesterone and set the transfer date. The GC will usually travel to the clinic a day or two before her transfer. The GC and IPs should discuss beforehand who will be in the room for the embryo transfer, but be aware that the clinic may have rules regarding the maximum number of people who may accompany her during the transfer. The transfer will occur, and she can go home the next day. Flying after a transfer does not seem to have a negative impact. After the transfer, the GC may remain close to home to complete her pregnancy testing and monitoring.

If they are pregnant, GCs continue to take medication per the clinic protocol until eight to twelve weeks gestational age. They will do their obstetrical ultrasounds with the transferring clinic (if local), the monitoring clinic, or their OB/GYN. Once the GC graduates from the fertility clinic, her care will be taken over by her local OB/GYN of choice. At that point, the fertility clinic fades into the background and waits hopefully for beautiful baby pictures.

Ideally, the GC has an uncomplicated pregnancy. The GC typically updates her IPs with progress. Some IPs go to clinic visits or ultrasounds, but most live in a different location and cannot regularly attend. Many GCs are very good about sending videos and updates, especially for important milestones. Some physicians may also video-conference appointments with the IPs.

As delivery approaches, travel plans for the IPs get more hectic. Some parents have the flexibility to travel to a location near the GC close to her due date and then stay until the baby can be brought home. Others plan to hop on a flight or get in the car as soon as labor starts. Most GCs are comfortable with having the parents in the room because they want the parents to share in the moment of birth. C-sections are different due to the restrictions of an operating room, but intended parents tend to be close by. Hopefully the hospital will accommodate the parents and give them a separate room where they can stay with the baby while the GC recovers. At this point, the relationship winds down as the parents take over their new responsibilities and begin working on the legal documentation necessary to bring their baby home.

We've said that in every fertility journey, it takes a village. In the case of gestational surrogacy, it requires more of a bustling small town! Clinics doing these cycles must have sufficient staff and knowledge to handle a case with so many moving parts. FDA rules, travel arrangements, and communication with multiple parties at once all factor into these complex journeys. They are not for the faint of heart, but the reward is incredible when a new little family joins the town.

CHAPTER 18

. . . .

LGBTQIA+
Family-Building

The universal human desire to create a family exists regardless of sex, sexual orientation, or gender identification. In general, the principles governing IVF remain the same independent of LGBTQIA+ status. That said, this population has additional considerations in treatment that may not apply to a cisgender, heteronormative population. From a medical perspective, a patient's current anatomy and hormonal status govern what treatments we can offer, as well as their partner (or lack thereof) and that person's current anatomy and hormonal status. Whether one or both partners were assigned female or male at birth influences their options to fulfill their dreams of family.

LET'S SPEAK THE
SAME LANGUAGE
· ·

Not everyone reading this book understands these terms, and we want all of our readers to get the most out of this. Here is a refresher on a limited list of terms:[1]

LGBTQIA+: lesbian, gay, bisexual, transgender, queer, questioning, intersex, asexual, and more (such as nonbinary, pansexual, etc.)

Sex: biological sex; refers to hormones, physiology, genes, and physical characteristics

Gender: a set of roles, activities, and behaviors a culture relates to an assigned sex

Orientation: sexual attraction to people or no one

AFAB: "assigned female at birth," a useful term to describe bodies with ovaries, tubes, and a uterus

AMAB: "assigned male at birth," a useful term to describe bodies with a penis, testicles, and scrotum

Asexual: not experiencing sexual attraction (sometimes shortened to "ace")

Heteronormative: the concept that everyone is attracted to the opposite sex, heterosexuality is the standard, and anything different is "abnormal"

Transgender: having a gender identity that does not match their sex at birth

Cisgender: having a gender identity that matches their sex at birth

CLINIC CHOICE

For any LGBTQIA+ patient, clinic choice is paramount in their comfort throughout this process. Not every clinic is open and affirming toward all patients. But the ones that are open to

LGBTQIA+ patients want nothing more and nothing less for you than they do for every patient: success in building your family in the most efficient and least traumatic way possible. Given our profession, there are relatively few things you can do or say to your physician that they have not experienced or heard before. Most centers working with LGBTQIA+ populations have little tolerance for team members who are not compassionate and comfortable with anyone who walks through the front door. We take extra care to ensure your desired pronouns and names are used. Despite good intentions, we may slip and use the wrong pronoun every now and then, particularly if your preferred name does not match your official documentation. Know that for official documentation in the medical record, we need to go by the name on your insurance card to ensure correct billing; the name on your driver's license is used to ensure that labeling on specimens is correct. Many name verifications occur between official documentation and our documentation to confirm correct specimens throughout the course of treatment.

RECIPROCAL IVF IN COUPLES, BOTH ASSIGNED FEMALE AT BIRTH (AFAB): TWO SETS OF EQUIPMENT

"Overwhelming" best describes the discussion surrounding an AFAB couple starting to consider their options for family-building. In fertility work, most of the time circumstances mean that we are backed into a corner in terms of treatment options. But in this situation we have the rare luxury of offering an abundance of choices for the couple to make.

If both halves of the couple possess both uterus and ovaries and are within specific age guidelines, they may choose multiple ways to participate. One option would be for one partner to provide eggs and the other one to provide the uterus. If there is a next pregnancy, the couple can then change roles, such that you are both a genetic parent and a gestational parent if desired. Another possibility would be for one partner to do both. Choices abound in this scenario!

Naturally, the same factors affecting fertility treatment success rates also apply in these cases. Age and health status greatly influence final decisions. If you are of advanced reproductive age, then you may not be the best one to provide eggs, regardless of your desire. Similarly, if you or your partner has a significant medical condition, it may not be appropriate to undergo the stress of a pregnancy.

Most patients in this situation are not infertile; however, some are. Sometimes diagnostic testing reveals issues in advance. Decreased ovarian reserve, damaged tubes, and uterine abnormalities frequently show up during the diagnostic phase. Unexplained infertility is trickier. Remember, in these cases, you may have normal results with no obvious problems. This means initial treatments may not work, causing severe angst and disappointment.

Social and psychological considerations often have a significant influence on treatment decisions. Frequently, one partner may feel a strong urge to carry the pregnancy, while the other partner may feel an equally strong urge *not* to carry the pregnancy. These preferences present challenges when medical indications push for a different decision. When the partner who wants to carry the pregnancy is not a good candidate, you must decide where priorities lie. Does it make more sense for the medically less-than-ideal partner to carry, taking the risk that may befall them or their child? Or does it make more sense for the partner who does not want to carry to take the responsibility, to make better health outcomes more likely? In some situations, the medical history dictates a decision.

For example, regardless of the patient's desire, most doctors decline to transfer an embryo to a patient with pulmonary hypertension because of the high risk of death. However, in a situation with a moderately hypertensive or diabetic patient compared to a healthy partner, the risk-benefit analysis may incorporate more factors than just the medical status. Individual values, shared values, medical facts, and personal preferences greatly influence decision-making and provide several layers of consideration for you. Decisions that seem obvious on paper become far more complex and nuanced in the context of the real world.

Divide and Conquer: Testing and Timing

One of the most significant advantages of reciprocal IVF is the ability to divide testing responsibilities. You both need physical exams and general lab work to ensure good health. Uterine- and ovarian-specific testing may be divvied up if you plan to share the burden of reproductive responsibilities. Fortunately, we don't much care about the uterus in a patient providing eggs unless it blocks our access to those eggs. On the flip side, the pregnant patient could have tiny shriveled-up raisins for ovaries and it won't change a thing.

Some couples elect for both partners to undergo fertility testing to compare results and make decisions based on achieving the best outcomes as a couple. This approach has advantages, particularly if both intend to contribute eggs and/or carry the pregnancies. We do discourage both partners from becoming pregnant at the exact same time. Pregnancy is a natural, happy event, but it is physically and emotionally taxing. Having two partners at the same stage of pregnancy presents logistical problems should complications arise. Similarly, two moms delivering close together means neither moms nor newborns have as much support available.

Concurrent testing allows for medical interventions to occur when necessary. For example, having a fibroid uterus can complicate an egg retrieval or transfer. Once the presence of fibroids is known, we can plan the necessary surgeries or procedures. During that time, your partner will start the IVF process. If your partner intends to retrieve eggs later but has diminished ovarian reserve, retrieving eggs now results in a better outcome even without an immediate embryo transfer. Testing both partners provides peace of mind and confidence in decision-making. If both intend to provide eggs and carry using the same sperm provider, you should consider additional testing. Checking CMV and carrier screening status on each partner early on ensures there is no potential mismatch.

FDA Testing and the Legalese

An intimate couple doing reciprocal IVF does not need certain parts of FDA testing. In these cases, the woman providing eggs is *not* considered an egg donor. The woman carrying the pregnancy is *not* considered a gestational carrier. You are simply considered a sexually intimate couple and intended parents. Sperm donors, on the other hand, are required to have FDA testing because they are not intimately related to the couple, nor are they going to have parental rights.

On a related topic, the need for legal contracts between parents doing reciprocal IVF varies widely. The laws that protect same-sex marriage do not extend to grant equal protection to same-sex parentage. Certain locations may make it difficult for same-sex parents to both be listed on a child's birth certificate. Additionally, even with a birth certificate, certain locations may not recognize the nonbiological parent as a parent. A consultation with a lawyer experienced in LGBTQIA+ parentage issues is always recommended. If a known donor is used, legal contracts between you and the donor are still necessary because this is a typical donor-recipient scenario. Contracts are already established if you obtain sperm from a cryobank.

DONOR-GC CYCLES IN PATIENTS
ASSIGNED MALE AT BIRTH (AMAB)

Single male parents, gay parents, and couples with both partners assigned male at birth (AMAB) have a tough road ahead of them. Given that they do not have direct ownership and jurisdiction over eggs or a uterus, they require much teamwork to build a family. Fortunately, all that teamwork is well supported and legal in the United States. However, just because surrogacy is not illegal in every state does not mean you want to jump into it. The state where your gestational carrier delivers is important. Some states have very unfavorable laws for same-sex male intended parents, or for same-sex male parents requiring a dual donor (both egg and sperm) situation. These states should be avoided. Other states have specifications regarding who may be an intended parent or a surrogate based on the status of marriage or relationship. This impacts what arrangements may be included in the agreement reached between intended parents and surrogate.

These issues are well worth researching before contracts are signed. Unfortunately, laws in the United States do not apply to the rest of the world, which is why a significant portion of LGBTQIA+ family-building occurs in the United States. Many American donors, clinics, and gestational carriers happily help these families, and a legal framework exists to make the process relatively seamless.

Cost considerations play a role with anyone pursuing fertility treatment, but they certainly hit harder in these couples, given the extensive support required to achieve success. Advance planning makes it more likely that you will achieve your desired family in a timely fashion. One way to decrease costs is to work with a known donor or look to a friend to participate as a gestational carrier. Another way to limit expense involves doing it right the first time. One thing definitely more expensive than a single IVF cycle is two cycles. Working with a cut-rate operation may seem like a good idea initially, but not if you must repeat the process after failing.

Deciding who will donate sperm to create embryos in a same-sex male couple also heavily influences costs in the process. A fresh donor cycle may produce a higher number of eggs. Still, no guarantee exists that you will obtain a high enough number of eggs for both sperm providers to have a good chance of creating genetically normal embryos. Finding proven egg donors helps mitigate this risk. Proven donors who both have high egg counts and meet donor selection criteria are difficult to find. Alternatively, buying multiple groups of frozen eggs guarantees the number of mature eggs, but it may cost more. Frozen eggs are convenient but undoubtedly require more than one group to achieve family goals with two different sperm providers. We know that, on average, approximately eight to ten mature eggs are likely needed to achieve one live birth. Unfortunately, with those estimates, just as with elective egg freezing, statistics work well when applied to ten thousand eggs but not terribly well when applied to ten eggs. There is no way to predict the number of embryos that will result in a given case.

In these cases, deciding on the number of embryos to obtain and the timing requires thought. Finding and screening a gestational carrier is time-consuming and expensive. If a couple has one embryo, that may be all they need to obtain a pregnancy and live birth. Problems occur if that embryo does not survive the thaw or result in a live birth. In those cases, we need to make more embryos, which starts the process again. You revert to finding a donor, obtaining eggs, creating embryos, and waiting for genetic testing results. The potential problem is that a GC may not want to wait for an extended period for that to be completed, particularly if a couple does not make decisions quickly. This scenario may require modification of the original contract with a gestational carrier, or new contracts to be prepared if a new gestational carrier must be found.

Creating multiple embryos before screening a GC turns out to be more cost-effective if the first transfer does not succeed. In this case, everyone moves quickly into a second attempt after a failed one. Obtaining more embryos from the outset costs more time and money up front. However, it may save you the time, expense, and hassle of finding a new gestational carrier later. The nuances in that decision revolve around the difficulty in creating embryos if other factors complicate the process. For example, poor sperm quality may have made the original embryo challenging to attain, which influences the decision about creating more embryos.

Due to the significant expense incurred during this process, many AMAB couples initially seek twin pregnancies via embryo transfers. Prior to the 2010s, as we've seen, multiple embryo transfers were common and even recommended due to much lower success rates. As success rates rose, the number of embryos to transfer decreased, and the focus shifted to improving the safety of pregnancies for both babies and the women who carried them. The biggest safety point in pregnancies involves avoiding multiple gestations. Today, gestational carriers are less willing to have multiple embryos transferred due to the increased risk, and clinics are less willing to transfer multiple embryos due to the known complications for all parties. As we noted in Chapter 1, many couples assume financial risk decreases with a double embryo transfer because it avoids the expense of a second transfer, but that is not the case. Twin pregnancies significantly increase costs due to complications of prematurity, time off work, advanced medical care, and double newborn and child expenses incurred at the same time.[2] The American College of Obstetricians and Gynecologists published a study showing that the increased cost of twins and triplets is not double or triple the cost of a single baby, but exponentially greater — four times and ten times the cost, respectively. Parents who have multiples also have a higher likelihood of stress, depression, relationship challenges, and impaired quality of life. Children of a multiple birth have a higher incidence of being the victims of child abuse.[3] Given the extremely high cost of multiples in so many areas of life, we try to avoid them when possible by doing single embryo transfers.

FDA TESTING CONSIDERATIONS

As mentioned previously, FDA testing occurs with all donor cycles. With anonymous egg and sperm donors, people who do not meet the donation criteria cannot become donors. When intended parents are the sperm providers, there is a higher likelihood that their sperm will not meet all the FDA criteria required for a donor. While this risk is avoidable when using a donor, it is unavoidable when an intended parent is the sperm provider. The GC must sign an acknowledgment of these risks. Reviewing the more common ones may alleviate some anxiety.

Two of the most commonly seen criteria that are not met in this particular situation include prior sexual relationships and living locations. Regarding the latter, recall that in 2016 Zika virus first emerged as a concern. Anyone who lived in an affected area had to have that risk factor delineated on their FDA forms. For better or worse, the entire globe was considered to be affected by Zika, and so for several years it surfaced on every eligibility form signed by GCs. Also, certain behaviors, such as multiple sexual partners or nonprescription injection drug use, are currently defined by the FDA as high-risk. As with all donations, communicable disease screening occurs before freezing specimens. The vast majority of the time, these tests are negative, making the "high-risk behavior" label relevant but mostly theoretical. Any positive test will be individually noted and discussed separately.

Intended parents who are actively sick or who have recently been sick don't tend to provide sperm samples due to decreased quality. But even if they were actively ill, the sperm is washed and separated from the seminal fluid before freezing at −80°C, and then individual sperm cells are picked up for direct injection into the egg before being placed in culture media that typically includes antibiotics. While it is always possible that a virus could be transmitted to a GC in this way, their risk is usually quite low. This particular discussion is especially relevant when talking about CMV antibodies, as discussed in Chapter 16 in the section on sperm donors; CMV does show up on the FDA risk form signed by the GC, though this ultimately poses much less risk to a GC than the pregnancy itself.

One idiosyncrasy of donors working with same-sex couples is that the donors are more frequently known to the intended parents. Often, this is because they are friends or family members who want to help their loved ones build their families. This is fantastic as long as a few principles are applied.

The first and arguably most important is ensuring the appropriate genetic boundaries. The two people providing egg and sperm cannot be blood relatives. This goes without saying, but sometimes when a completely unrelated person is carrying the pregnancy, it is easier to forget the obvious. A core consideration is avoiding the appearance of impropriety. For example, a carrying mom using her brother as a sperm donor with her partner's egg has no genetic concerns. It is worth making it clear to any other family members that there was no improper relationship between the sister and brother involved. While caring what others think is not important, the possibility of appearing to have broken a major social taboo is worth considering.

The second consideration is the greater world and how these relationships function outside of parentage concerns. The last thing anyone wants is for a loved one to think their donation will be the only way they will be acknowledged by the intended parents or children. On the other hand, it is of paramount importance for the intended parent to avoid coercion, either intentional or unintentional. A situation in which a mother is asking to use her daughter's eggs to create a family with a new partner must be evaluated closely due to power dynamics in a parent-child relationship. This does not mean it may not be the right thing to do, but it is well worth additional attention.

Disclosure of these genetic relationships to the resulting children is incredibly important. Children of non-heteronormative couples are unlikely to be surprised by the information that their parents needed help conceiving. Still, it is important that children know about their origins from an early age to maintain a trusting, dynamic relationship between parents and children and avoid bombshells being dropped at holiday dinners.

TRANS PATIENTS

In general, the techniques and success rates of fertility treatment with trans patients mirror those of cisgender patients. Treatments available to you will depend upon your reproductive organs and the current status of those organs. A patient who has already completed gender-affirming surgery in the form of hysterectomy and oophorectomy will have a very different role than a trans man who has a uterus and ovaries, with or without gender-affirming hormonal therapy.

A trans patient currently undergoing hormonal therapy can generally provide eggs or sperm for family-building. A bigger question is whether they want to do so. This is a personal decision and depends on several conditions. They may have to stop gender-affirming hormonal therapy and may need to undergo additional treatment to obtain their gametes. Trans women taking estrogen may or may not still be making sperm. If they are still making sperm, collecting and using that sperm is fairly straightforward. If they are not, it may be necessary to stop estrogen treatment and begin medication to encourage sperm production. Sperm production may resume in the testes in as little as three months, but it may take much longer; more data is needed in this area.[4] Whether or not a patient chooses to undergo this treatment depends on their tolerance for hormones, mentally and physically.

A trans man desiring to give eggs for family-building must undergo more extensive treatment in the form of egg retrieval. They may or may not continue their testosterone while undergoing ovarian stimulation, depending on their physician's comfort level and the evolution of research in this area (as an example, many patients with PCOS have naturally high levels of testosterone and have good results after IVF). Many physicians prefer for trans men to stop their testosterone in the midst of stimulation, but it is for a relatively short period of time and should not impact ultimate pregnancy rates.[5] The more concerning issue for trans men is the constant reminder of their female reproductive organs. During treatment, they need transvaginal ultrasounds and an increase in female reproductive hormones during the stimulation cycle. The use of medications like letrozole to keep estrogen levels low may help, but that does not negate the need for frequent vaginal ultrasounds and a vaginal oocyte retrieval.

Trans men who have undergone hysterectomy and trans women may need to work with a GC to carry a pregnancy if their partner is unable to do so. Trans men who still have a uterus and desire to carry the pregnancy may do so after stopping their gender-affirming hormones.[6] Elevated levels of testosterone negatively impact the growing fetus, but limited data suggests that children of trans men who stopped their testosterone during pregnancy have reassuring outcomes.[7]

―――――――

This is just a peek into the world of LGBTQIA+ family-building. Each family's needs are unique, and we are honored, and grateful, to be a part of a technology that can truly help build every and any family.

. . . .

CHAPTER 19

Beyond Infertility: The Other Reasons for Choosing IVF

A couple of decades ago, the only reason to do IVF was for infertility. A woman with blocked tubes or a man with a very low sperm count could not get pregnant without the lab physically putting the egg and sperm together. The technology was incredible in 1978 when Louise Brown was the first IVF baby born in England. Today, almost unbelievable advances in other areas of genetics and medicine have widely expanded the ways IVF improves patients' lives.

RECURRENT PREGNANCY LOSS: IMPROVING THE ODDS

Many couples do IVF to improve pregnancy success rates. Patients with recurrent pregnancy loss do not have difficulty conceiving but have challenges staying pregnant. Recurrent pregnancy loss affects up to 2–4 percent of women of reproductive age. Women who have already experienced two or three pregnancy losses have a 30 percent chance of another loss, and medical evaluation may help prevent another devastating experience.[1] Many women with recurrent pregnancy loss choose to do IVF to help improve their odds of a successful conception.

Doing IVF improves the odds by transferring a genetically normal embryo using preimplantation genetic testing for aneuploidy (PGT-A). We know that approximately 25 to 50 percent of all miscarriages occur because the baby has aneuploidy (too few or too many chromosomes as a result of random sorting errors in the egg).[2] If we transfer a chromosomally normal embryo, we change the tipping point, and pregnancies in these patients continue to full term more often. Ensuring that the embryo contains 46 chromosomes greatly improves the odds of a live birth by significantly decreasing the possibility of implantation of an abnormal embryo, but it cannot guarantee that outcome because so many other factors go into the development of a healthy baby. As genetic technology improves, we may even find genes responsible for miscarriage within the embryo itself, such as abnormal genes that prevent the growth of the placenta or cause early changes in vital organs like the tiny fetal heart.

In some cases, the abnormal number of chromosomes in the embryo is not a random accident. As we saw in Chapter 11, when an adult with a balanced translocation (a scrambling of DNA that occurred when that person was an embryo) tries to conceive, the chromosomes in their sperm or eggs won't divide in an exact 50/50 split, which will result in an embryo with the wrong number of chromosomes. PGT-SR will locate and identify these imbalances prior to implantation, improving live birth rates.

A more perplexing question is whether or not IVF will help improve the outcome for couples with unexplained recurrent pregnancy loss. In about 50 percent of couples who have experienced recurrent pregnancy loss, no identifiable reason for those losses has been found.[3] The hormonal, anatomic, and potential inherited genetic causes have been eliminated. That frustrates all of us, as we want nothing more than to identify the problem and fix it immediately. For many couples, it is hard to keep trying to conceive after multiple miscarriages. At some point, most patients and their docs start talking about IVF.

The benefit of IVF for couples with recurrent miscarriages is recognized. Recent data suggests that IVF does improve the odds of a successful pregnancy, even in couples with recurrent miscarriages.[4] One possible source of benefit is the tight control of the hormonal environment for your embryo during IVF. This includes pH-balanced, temperature-controlled, environmentally regulated culture media. Growing your embryos for a few days in our lab makes them hardier and more likely to develop inside your uterus. Our tight control extends to the uterine environment as well. As described in earlier chapters, we examine the cavity thoroughly shortly before transfer if needed, to ensure no inflammation or structural abnormalities exist. We then monitor it meticulously as it develops under carefully curated hormonal input. Using medications allows us to influence endometrial development in ways that may not be occurring naturally, thereby improving the chance of a successful pregnancy.

GENETICS: AN OUNCE OF PREVENTION IS WORTH A POUND OF CURE

Genetic techniques have evolved to examine as many parts of the DNA as possible, and some future parents want or need that information prior to conceiving. Today we look at all 23 pairs of chromosomes in every embryo, and improvements in technology allow us to get far more accurate details about each chromosome than was possible in the past. And the technology continues to improve: Recently, the company Genomic Prediction developed a way to evaluate 1.6 million areas on the DNA of each chromosome, making the results even more precise.

PGT-A

When women are over thirty-five years of age, their risk of bearing a child with chromosomal abnormalities starts to increase. Such abnormalities often significantly impact the life of the child. As we saw in Chapter 11, Down syndrome, when there are three copies of chromosome 21, is a widely known example of this. There are other abnormalities, such as an extra copy of chromosome 13 or 18, that are more common in older women, and babies born with these abnormalities will have a devastatingly short lifespan. Women who want to minimize the risk of a pregnancy that will result in the birth of a medically complex child turn to IVF with PGT-A to identify those abnormalities prior to implantation.

PGT-M

Other couples do IVF to prevent their baby from developing a life-threatening genetic condition. Most of us carry at least one "bad" gene but are not affected by the condition because we have a corresponding normal gene, so having one of these abnormal genes is usually problematic only if you and your partner carry the exact same ones. Thankfully, fertility doctors routinely check carrier screening tests before fertility treatments. But because companies who do such screening are adding more genes to their panels every few years, if you had this test done several years ago we recommend that both you and your partner get the newest version.

About 1 in 550 couples test positive for the same deleterious gene. And it's not always the case that this happens in couples who come from very similar ethnic backgrounds or are distantly related. Your genetic makeup can be surprising. Unrelated patients of different ethnic backgrounds may test positive for the same unique condition. The only way to know if you and your partner carry one of these conditions is by doing an expanded carrier screening test before you do IVF. It may cost a few hundred dollars, but the results are priceless if you are part of a carrier couple. This information prevents your child from getting a terrible disease. If you test positive, don't hide the news in the closet like an ugly Christmas sweater; let your family know, as the knowledge you've discovered may save a future niece, nephew, or cousin.

If you and your partner carry the same recessive gene or if one of you carries a dominant gene, genetic counseling helps you understand the significance of your results. All expanded carrier screening companies offer genetic counseling as part of the cost. Fertility docs can help you decide whether you should do genetic testing on your embryos. But we do not know the details of each condition. Genetic counselors give you specific information about genetic conditions and their impact on your future child. Often, after genetic counseling, couples are shocked to learn about the severity of the disease they carry a gene for, even though they have no symptoms. Most often, partners choose to do genetic testing rather than take the chance of having an affected child. However, that is not the case for all. In some situations, carrier couples discover they have a milder form of an abnormal gene, which may not cause significant difficulties in their future child. They may also decide to test the child shortly after birth to ensure the baby gets an early intervention to improve the outcome.

Remember our discussion in Chapter 10 of how IVF is a numbers game? If you are under thirty-five and have a good egg number, you may get ten to fifteen eggs at the time of egg retrieval, but ultimately, you may end up with only three to six embryos to test with PGT-A. Statistically, about half of your embryos will have the correct number of chromosomes, resulting in two to three genetically normal embryos available for transfer in an average retrieval. If you are thirty-six or older your outcome may not be as good, meaning fewer (if any) genetically normal embryos.

Only embryos with the correct number of chromosomes are evaluated further for single gene abnormalities, which are genetic conditions caused by an abnormality in a single gene. If the condition is recessive, the good news is that on average, 75 percent of the remaining embryos will not be affected by the gene — half of the embryos will be a carrier, just like you, and 25 percent will have no abnormal genes — but 25 percent will carry both abnormal genes. In these situations, the egg number becomes even more critical than usual. The more eggs you get, the more likely you will have a normal embryo without the genetic condition. It is like lottery tickets—the more you buy, the better your chances are. In this case, it is not unusual to do IVF at least twice to complete your family, given the challenge of creating a healthy embryo.

Other genes are inherited as autosomal dominant. They can be inherited from the mother or father. If a gene is inherited in that way, the presence of only one copy results in the abnormal condition. Approximately 50 percent of offspring will inherit the abnormal gene. Achondroplasia dwarfism is an example of an autosomal dominant gene.

In some cases, the problematic gene is tied to a sex chromosome — the X or Y chromosome that determines the sex of the baby. This is called a sex-linked trait. Patients who know this may elect to avoid using PGT-M with its greater expense and complexity, and instead choose to avoid transferring embryos of the affected sex. An example of this would be types of muscular dystrophy (a severe condition that leads to muscles wasting away) that are tied to the X chromosome. Males have only one X chromosome, so if this chromosome is affected, the child will be affected by the disease. There is a 50/50 chance of the male embryo getting the affected chromosome. Females have two X chromosomes, so a female child may carry the disease but not be affected. In this example, families carrying sex-linked traits do not transfer male embryos so as to avoid a child affected by muscular dystrophy.

PGT-P

As discussed in Chapter 11, a new technology called PGT-P looks at multiple genes that cause problems in your future baby. PGT-P predicts which of your embryos is more likely to be impacted by adult diseases. This test does not concretely identify which embryos will be affected by a given disease, but it can identify which embryo from a grouping may be at the lowest risk for that condition. Diseases evaluated with PGT-P include type 1 and type 2 diabetes, breast cancer, schizophrenia, melanoma, heart disease, and high blood pressure. Many of these conditions are associated with more than one gene. At present only a few fertility centers do PGT-P, but stay tuned as we learn more about the inheritance of complicated diseases. This new genetic technology may be part of a couple's genetic choice if they decide to do IVF. In the future, we may be able to predict which embryo is more likely to survive and thrive by analyzing genes regulating embryo development.

THIRD-PARTY REPRODUCTION

One important reason couples pursue IVF is a need for additional help in building their family for health and safety reasons. Help may come in the form of a sperm, egg, or embryo donor, or a gestational carrier (who carries the pregnancy but is not biologically related to the child). If a woman has severe heart or lung disease, for example, getting pregnant may have an extremely high mortality rate. She may need a gestational carrier to carry the pregnancy for her. Alternatively, some people affected by both significant genetic conditions and lower egg or sperm supplies may require an egg, sperm, or embryo donor. Doing so allows them to get pregnant without their child being affected by the severe disease they carry. We explore this world in great detail in Chapters 16, 17, and 18.

SPIN CYCLE: BUILDING A FAMILY FAST

One of the great advantages of modern medicine is the ability to carry out advanced testing that identifies diseases before they become severe, debilitating, or deadly. Some patients need IVF because they are facing development of a more severe disease with an effective treatment that would negatively impact their fertility. Inherited cancer syndromes like BRCA particularly impact young women because the treatment to avoid developing ovarian cancer involves removing the ovaries while they are relatively young, potentially before childbearing is completed or even started. In other instances, women with precancerous cells of the uterus may require hysterectomy in the relatively near future — they have time to have their own children, but they cannot afford to wait for a pregnancy to happen spontaneously. In these cases, IVF may allow them to create embryos quickly, expediting the process of receiving more definitive treatment for their underlying health condition.

FAMILY PLANNING AND
FAMILY BALANCING

You may strongly desire multiple children but were not ready to pursue creating a family until an older age, perhaps after meeting a partner, becoming financially stable, graduating from school, or moving to a certain location. This delay in childbearing would be unlikely to seriously hinder your ability to have a first child but is highly likely to impair your ability to have more than one child. In these cases, you may opt for IVF to bank embryos. This way, even though you may not be ready for your second child until you are forty-three years old, you have embryos from when you were thirty-six years old. With embryos originating from younger eggs, the chance of a second live birth is considerably higher.

Other patients will have preferences for sex selection in their embryos. You may strongly desire male or female children in a specific order. The only reliable way to achieve this information is through IVF with PGT-A. We cannot guarantee you will get an embryo of the desired sex, but we can transfer an embryo of the desired sex if we get one.

In this chapter, we discussed why you may want to do IVF even if getting pregnant is not a problem for you and your partner. As we discussed, genetic testing can prevent your child from inheriting debilitating or deadly genes. It may decrease the chance of having multiple miscarriages for couples with recurrent pregnancy loss. It is a valuable tool in family planning and family balancing, as well as shortening the time to delivery in cases of medical necessity. In the future, more couples may use IVF to prevent conditions resulting from inheriting a certain gene group. As medicine evolves, more conditions can be evaluated and treated in the embryology lab, preventing significant pain and suffering.

AFTERWORD

Going through infertility care, especially IVF, can be one of the hardest but most rewarding journeys of your life. We hope that through *The IVF Blueprint* we have helped give you the information you need to build the family of your dreams through the science and miracle of IVF. Knowledge is power, and with the tools we have provided, you are well prepared for the journey ahead.

There are many intricacies to the art of in vitro fertilization. And though we cannot give you direct guidance for every scenario and situation, we know that you can do this. Always remember that your REI specialist and clinical team are *your* team, and you are not in this alone. We are rooting for *you*!

Your Fertility Docs Uncensored,
Abby, Carrie, and Susan

ACKNOWLEDGMENTS

···

Writing this book has been a wild ride, and it wouldn't have been possible without a small army of incredible humans cheering us on.

To the listeners of *Fertility Docs Uncensored,* this book exists because of you. Your bravery in sharing your stories turned what could have been a lonely road into a vibrant, supportive community. You're the reason we've spent countless hours behind microphones — and now on these pages. Thank you for being the heartbeat of everything we do.

Our thanks go to the rock star team at Hachette, including Michael Szczerban, the masterly VP and publisher of Little, Brown Spark, and our editor extraordinaire, Cara Bedick, who somehow managed to juggle three opinionated authors with finesse. And to Regina Ryan, our fearless literary agent — you believed in us as first-time authors and understood why this book is needed. To all the behind-the-scenes magicians who made this project a reality, we're endlessly grateful.

A huge shout-out to our sponsors and the team behind *Fertility Docs Uncensored.* Without your belief in our mission (and your financial support), we wouldn't have made it to over three hundred episodes and more than a million downloads. Special thanks to Amy Hall and the Catalyst team, including Brandy Thomas, for the genius idea to launch the podcast in March 2020 and for guiding us through the chaos. Cheryl Bemis, thanks for making us feel like supermodels during our photo shoots. Five years of fun, growth, and unforgettable memories — we couldn't have done it without you.

Much gratitude to our partners in crime at US Fertility, Ovation Fertility, Progyny, California Cryobank, Seattle Sperm Bank, Form Health, Needed, and Alife Health. We hugely appreciate Dr. Mark Ratner, medical director of Theralogix, for sharing his encyclopedic knowledge of supplements, and Tiffany Graham, MPH, RDN, LDN, for the invaluable articles sent for the supplements chapter. Katherine Provost, Esq., your succinct legal advice regarding the complicated third-party reproduction chapters made us swoon. Dr. Tex VerMilyea, your lab expertise is appreciated a dozen times daily, and now in the lab chapters. We also appreciate Chris Jackson, president of Cicero Diagnostics, and his colleague Dan Angress. Dr. Kristen Brogaard, Lauren Burleson, and Andy Olson from Path Fertility, we appreciate your support and knowledge. Thank you for helping us keep the lights on and the dream alive.

To our families — thank you for loving, feeding, and tolerating us while we obsessed over this project. Here are our individual acknowledgments:

From Abby:
Rick, from the day we met in Gainesville, you have been my greatest source of love and support. Now we've built a beautiful life and family together. Thank you for being my partner in every sense of the word — for sharing laughter and love and doing all the laundry and cooking dinner as I chased my dreams. You are my greatest blessing and my home.

To my children, Benjamin and Hailey, you are the most unexpected and precious gifts of my life. I am so proud of you both. I cannot wait to see what you accomplish. Going through IVF was difficult but well worth the challenge since it gave me you. I can see now that the journey turned out to be a blessing in disguise since it made me a better mom, doctor, and person.

Bobby and Charles Eblen, thank you for the love and encouragement that shaped me. Mom, you were a trailblazer and inspiration — a chemist at a time when few women had a degree. I miss you so much. And to my sister, Lee Aikens — thank you for always believing in me (even if I'm still holding a grudge about that snowball).

To my mentors, Vivian Newman (best biology teacher ever, who taught me frog IVF), Patrick Duff, MD, Steve Nakajima, MD, Christine Cook, MD, and Marvin Yussman, MD — thank you for your wisdom and guidance. I also thank Dr. Donna Vogel, the first REI specialist I met, who let me work as a college student with her at the NIH. And to my colleagues at Nashville Fertility Center — George Hill, MD, Christine Whitworth, MD, Glenn Weitzman, MD, Kristin Van Heertum, MD, Meghan Smith, MD, and Meredith Humphreys, MD — you are an incredible team and a joy to work with. Thanks to our nurses and clinical support staff, who are always at the top of their game and provide great support for our infertility patients.

Finally, to my lifelong friends: Jeanie Crotts, my college roommate, who never stopped pushing me to get more involved in college activities; Kellee Dicks, who welcomed me to her Louisville tribe when I did not know anyone; Karen Pompeo, Jan Beach, Ellen Henley, Daphne Bright, Shelley Ozdil, whom I am so happy to have found in college and who provide great entertainment on our Sigma Kappa girls' trips; Susie Fleming, Angie Moore, Sarah Cronan, Julie Turner, and Chris Rogers, who have been my besties since middle school (I'm so lucky to have you); Annette Kyzer, MD, and Cathy Thornburg, MD, who invited me into your circle when I came to Nashville, and whose friendship I cherish; Robin Hansel, whose literary advice and encouragement are pure gold. Thank you all for being my people.

From Carrie:

To my husband, Dr. Mark Dugan, I love you more than chocolate. You are my biggest cheerleader, my favorite person, and the best choice I ever made. Words cannot express my joy in spending life with you.

To Ava and Jack, you bring constant smiles and are growing up to be such lovely human beings. I look forward to every day with you. I will never stop asking "Do you know how much I love you?" with the forever reply "All the amounts."

To moooooooooommm, Mary Bedient, you take such good care of me, I love you. I am here because you were there.

To dad Jack, and bonus dad Ron, the most patient humans I know, I miss you both. Your love of everything educational lives on.

To my in-laws, John, Dena, Marissa, Jon, Gracie, and Melina, I love you bunches. Dena, thank you for your help with all the questions as we were getting this project started.

To my tribe, Adele Powers, Dr. Michelle Young, Dr. Eve Ringsmuth, Sarah Stout, Dr. Jeremy O'Brien, Drs. Megan and Scott Cheney, Drs. Jenn Parod and Steve Howell, Drs. Veneta George and Chris Murray, Serge and Melissa Depelchin, Marcie and Dr. Morgan Pomeranz, I appreciate your wit, your brilliance, your creativity, your practicality, your good humor, your insights, and most of all the joy and love you bring into my life.

To my family at the Fertility Center of Las Vegas, I feel so lucky to have found all of you. Dr. Bruce Shapiro, your unwavering support and faith in me mean the world. Dr. Leah Kaye, I am so lucky to have such a brilliant, kind, delightful person in the office next door every day. To Forest Garner, thank you for always making me think, even against my will. To Shelley Schulte and Kim Trede, your sunny smiles and immaculate organization keep me together and I am so incredibly grateful. To every single other member of the team, singing your praises would be a book unto itself. I am grateful to have you all by my side every day, unfailing in your dedication to taking care of our patients.

Dr. Donna Session and Dr. Jessica Spencer, I still hear your voices in my ears. Dr. Jenn Kawwass and Dr. Heather Hipp, I am fortunate to have trained with you. Dr. Jeffrey Goldberg, thank you for introducing me to the world of REI and giving me the boost to get here.

To my proofreader patients, I am so grateful for your help. To all my patients, your thirst for knowledge and understanding to help you build your families inspires me daily.

From Susan:

To my husband, Brook: Thank you for being my partner, best friend, and steadfast companion through every twist and turn life has offered us over these past thirty years. I am endlessly grateful for you, and I love you with all my heart.

To my children, Beck, Blaine, and Brynn: You are my greatest blessings and three of the most incredible people I know. Thank you for loving me as much as I love you — you fill my life with joy and pride every single day.

To my parents, Minnie and Charlie: Your unwavering love and belief in me taught me that I could accomplish anything my heart and mind desired. I carry your love and lessons with me every day.

To Thomas Wincek, MD, and Charles Coddington, MD: Thank you for seeing my potential and guiding me toward the extraordinary world of REI. Your faith in me has shaped my career and changed my life forever.

To my colleagues at Texas Fertility Center: Thank you for supporting the launch of the podcast and for your constant encouragement. To Kaylen Silverberg, MD: Your encouragement and support, especially when I think outside the box, mean more to me than words can express. To Erika Munch, MD: Your friendship, insight,

and brilliance as an editor and colleague have been invaluable —
having you by my side is a true blessing. To Sandra McCready:
Thank you for everything you do. Your dedication and positivity
brighten every day and make a lasting difference!

To Brandy: Thank you for always being a source of support.
Your friendship is truly priceless, and I'm so lucky to have you.

To Kelsey: Thank you for your faith in my vision. Your friendship is a gift I treasure deeply.

To Erin: Thank you for your friendship, warm hugs, and for
always being there to listen. Your kindness and presence mean
everything to me.

To Helle: Even across an ocean, we've remained amazing
friends. I love you and your family so much, and I can't wait for our
next adventure together!

To Dilyn: Thank you for trusting me. You are a force of nature
and a dear friend, and I'm so grateful for you.

To Krista: You are an incredible person. Thank you for allowing
me to be part of your journey — it's an honor to be your friend.

And, of course, to you, dear reader: Whether you're navigating
infertility, supporting someone who is, or just curious, thank you
for picking up this book. Your courage and resilience are why this
work matters. Here's to the journey, the laughter, and the stories
that unite us.

NOTES
. . . .

CHAPTER 1 — WHAT YOU NEED TO KNOW ABOUT IVF BEFORE YOU START

1. Practice Committee of the American Society for Reproductive Medicine, "Evidence-Based Treatments for Couples with Unexplained Infertility: A Guideline," *Fertility and Sterility* 113, no. 2 (2020): 305–322.

2. Practice Committee of the American Society for Reproductive Medicine, "Evidence-Based Treatments."

3. E. V. Lemos et al., "Healthcare Expenses Associated with Multiple vs Singleton Pregnancies in the United States," *American Journal of Obstetrics and Gynecology* 209 (2013): 586:e1–e11.

4. American College of Obstetricians and Gynecologists, "Multifetal Pregnancy Reduction: Committee Opinion No. 719," *Obstetrics and Gynecology* 130 (2017): e158–e163.

CHAPTER 2 — DECIDING ON IVF: THE KEY QUESTIONS AND THE FIRST STEPS

1. A. Uglietti et al., "The Risk of Malignancy in Uterine Polyps: A Systematic Review and Meta-Analysis," *European Journal of Obstetrics, Gynecology, and Reproductive Biology* 237 (2019): 48–56, DOI: 10.1016/j.ejogrb.2019.04.009.

2. M. T. Sauerbrun-Cutler et al., "Is Intracytoplasmic Sperm (ICSI) Better than Traditional In Vitro Fertilization (IVF): Confirmation of Higher Blastocyst Rates per Oocyte Using a Split Insemination Design," *Journal of Assisted Reproduction and Genetics* 37, no. 7 (2020): 1661–1667, DOI: 10.1007/s10815-020-01819-1.

3. A. D. Domar, "The Psychological Impact of Infertility: A Comparison with Patients and Other Medical Conditions," *Journal of Psychosomatic Obstetrics & Gynaecology* 14 Suppl. (1993): 45–52.

CHAPTER 4 — GETTING READY FOR IVF: IT'S LIKE BUILDING A HOUSE

1. D. L. Hoyert, "Maternal Mortality Rates in the United States, 2021," NCHS Health E-Stats, 2023, https://dx.doi.org/10.15620/cdc:124678.

2. Centers for Disease Control and Prevention, "Pregnancy Mortality Surveillance System," March 23, 2023, https://www.cdc.gov/reproductivehealth/maternal-mortality/pregnancy-mortality-surveillance-system.htm.

3. Centers for Disease Control and Prevention, "Pregnant? Don't Overlook Blood Clots," February 12, 2020, https://www.cdc.gov/ncbddd/dvt/features/blood-clots-pregnant-women.html; T. T. Lao, "Pulmonary Embolism in Pregnancy and the Puerperium," *Best Practice and Research: Clinical Obstetrics & Gynaecology* 85, pt. A (2022): 96–106, DOI: 10.1016/j.bpobgyn.2022.06.003.

4. Centers for Disease Control and Prevention, "Pregnancy Mortality Surveillance System."

5. A. P. MacKay et al., "Pregnancy-Related Mortality from Preeclampsia and Eclampsia," *Obstetrics and Gynecology* 97, no. 4 (2001): 533–538.

6. S. R. Martin and A. Edwards, "Pulmonary Hypertension and Pregnancy," *Obstetrics and Gynecology* 134, no. 5 (2019): 974–987, DOI:10.1097/AOG.0000000000003549.

7. N. U. Chowdhury et al., "Sex and Gender in Asthma," *European Respiratory Review* 30, no. 162 (2021): 210067, DOI 10.1183/16000617.0067-2021.

8. J. E. Dominguez et al., "Management of Obstructive Sleep Apnea in Pregnancy," *Obstetrics and Gynecology Clinics of North America* 45, no. 2 (2018): 233–247, DOI: 10.1016/j.ogc.2018.01.001.

9. J. Bennett et al., "Spinal Cord Injuries," StatPearls, 2023, https://www.ncbi.nlm.nih.gov/books/NBK560721/.

10. Y. Wang et al., "Multiple Sclerosis and Pregnancy: Pathogenesis, Influencing Factors, and Treatment Options," *Autoimmunity Reviews* 22, no. 11 (2023): 103449, DOI: 10.1016/j.autrev.2023.103449.

11. G. Varytė et al., "Pregnancy and Multiple Sclerosis: An Update," *Current Opinion in Obstetrics and Gynecology* 33, no. 5 (2021): 378–383, DOI: 10.1097/GCO.0000000000000731.

12. S. Y. Gao et al., "Selective Serotonin Reuptake Inhibitor Use During Early Pregnancy and Congenital Malformations: A Systematic Review and Meta-Analysis of Cohort Studies of More than 9 Million Births," *BMC Medicine* 16, no. 1 (2018): 205, DOI: 10.1186/s12916-018-1193-5.

13. H. Lee et al., "Pregnancy and Neonatal Outcomes After Exposure to Alprazolam in Pregnancy," *Frontiers in Pharmacology* 13 (2022): 854562, DOI: 10.3389/fphar.2022.854562.

14. A. G. Jensen et al., "Prenatal Exposure to Benzodiazepines and the Development of the Offspring—A Systematic Review," *Neurotoxicology and Teratology* 91 (2022): 107078, DOI: 10.1016/j.ntt.2022.107078.

15. "Treatment and Management of Mental Health Conditions During Pregnancy and Postpartum: ACOG Clinical Practice Guideline No. 5," *Obstetrics and Gynecology* 141, no. 6 (2023): 1262–1288, DOI: 10.1097/AOG.0000000000005202.

16. A. Rogers et al., "Association Between Maternal Perinatal Depression and Anxiety and Child and Adolescent Development: A Meta-analysis," *JAMA Pediatrics* 174, no. 11 (2020): 1082–1092, DOI: 10.1001/jamapediatrics.2020.2910.

17. J. Bustamante, "NCDAS: Substance Abuse and Addiction Statistics," 2023, NCDAS, https://drugabusestatistics.org.

18. U. Mahadevan et al., "Inflammatory Bowel Disease in Pregnancy Clinical Care Pathway: A Report from the American Gastroenterological Association IBD Parenthood Project Working Group," *Gastroenterology* 156, no. 5 (2019): 1508–1524, DOI: 10.1053/j.gastro.2018.12.022.

19. K. Arvanitakis et al., "Adverse Pregnancy Outcomes in Women with Celiac Disease: A Systematic Review and Meta-Analysis," *Annals of Gastroenterology* 36, no. 1 (2023): 12–24, DOI: 10.20524/aog.2022.0764.

20. Centers for Disease Control and Prevention, National Diabetes Statistics Report website, https://www.cdc.gov/diabetes/data/statistics-report/index.html, accessed November 29, 2023.

21. Y. Shen et al., "Gestational Diabetes with Diabetes and Prediabetes Risks: A Large Observational Study," *European Journal of Endocrinology* 179, no. 1 (2018): 51–58, DOI: 10.1530/EJE-18-0130.

22. J. H. Moon and H. C. Jang, "Gestational Diabetes Mellitus: Diagnostic Approaches and Maternal-Offspring Complications," *Diabetes and Metabolism Journal* 46, no. 1 (2022): 3–14, DOI: 10.4093/dmj.2021.0335.

CHAPTER 5 — LIFESTYLE CHANGES THAT BENEFIT MOM AND BABY

1. V. Layoun et al., "Pregnancy Outcomes Associated with the Use of Tobacco and Marijuana," *Clinical Obstetrics & Gynecology* 65 (2022): 376–387.

2. Layoun et al., "Pregnancy Outcomes Associated with the Use of Tobacco and Marijuana."

3. J. R. Whittington et al., "The Use of Electronic Cigarettes in Pregnancy: A Review of the Literature," *Obstetrical and Gynecological Survey* 73, no. 9 (2018): 544–549.

4. S. Sarrafpour et al., "Considerations and Implications of Cannabidiol Use During Pregnancy," *Current Pain and Headache Reports* 24, no. 7 (2020): 38, https://doi.org/10.1007/s11916-020-00872.

5. G. I. Martin, "Marijuana: The Effects on Pregnancy, the Fetus, and the Newborn," *Journal of Perinatology* 40 (2020): 1470–1476.

6. J. Friedrich et al., "The Grass Isn't Always Greener: The Effects of Cannabis on Embryological Development," *BMC Pharmacology and Toxicology* 17 (2016): 45.

7. Martin, "Marijuana: The Effects on Pregnancy, the Fetus, and the Newborn."

8. American Society for Reproductive Medicine and American College of Obstetricians and Gynecologists, "Committee Opinion 162: Prepregnancy Counseling," *Fertility and Sterility* 111, no. 1 (2022): 32–42.

9. S. C. Langley-Evans et al., "Overweight, Obesity and Excessive Weight Gain in Pregnancy as Risk Factors for Adverse Pregnancy Outcomes: A Narrative Review," *Journal of Human Nutrition Dietetics* 35 (2022): 250–264.

10. P. Liu et al., "Association Between Perinatal Outcomes and Maternal Pre-Pregnancy Body Mass Index," *Obesity Reviews* 17, no. 11 (2016): 1091–1102, https://doi.org/10.1111/obr.12455.

11. E. A. Day et al., "Metformin-Induced Increases in GDF15 Are Important for Suppressing Appetite and Promoting Weight Loss," *Nature Metabolism* 1, no. 12 (2019): 1202–1208, DOI: 10.1038/s42255-019-0146-4.

12. R. J. Griffith et al., "Interventions to Prevent Women from Developing Gestational Diabetes Mellitus: An Overview of Cochrane Reviews," *Cochrane Database of Systematic Reviews* 6, no. 6 (2020): CD012394, DOI: 10.1002/14651858.CD012394.pub3.

13. B. M. Nørgård et al., "Adverse Birth and Child Outcomes in Children Fathered by Men Treated with Antidiabetics Prior to Conception: A Nationwide Cohort Study," *Journal of Clinical Medicine* 11, no. 21 (2022): 6595, DOI: 10.3390/jcm11216595.

14. National Center for Biotechnology Information, "PubChem Compound Summary for CID 4771, Phentermine," accessed December 11, 2023, https://pubchem.ncbi.nlm.nih.gov/compound/Phentermine.

15. M. Bossart et al., "Effects on Weight Loss and Glycemic Control with SAR441255, a Potent Unimolecular Peptide GLP-1/GIP/GCG Receptor Triagonist," *Cell Metabolism* 34, no. 1 (2022): 59–74.e10, DOI: 10.1016/j.cmet.2021.12.005.

16. American Society for Reproductive Medicine and American College of Obstetricians and Gynecologists, "Committee Opinion 162: Prepregnancy Counseling."

17. R. Barakat et al., "Exercise During Pregnancy Is Associated with a Shorter Duration of Labor: A Randomized Clinical Trial," *European Journal of Obstetrics, Gynecology, and Reproductive Biology* 224 (2018): 33–40, https://doi.org/10.1016/j.ejogrb.2018.03.009.

18. J. L. Oei, "Alcohol Use in Pregnancy and Its Impact on the Mother and Child," *Addiction* 115 (2020): 2148–2163.

19. K. K. Keshav et al., "An Update on Fetal Alcohol Syndrome — Pathogenesis, Risks, and Treatment," *Alcoholism: Clinical and Experimental Research* 40, no. 8 (2016): 1594–1602.

20. American Society for Reproductive Medicine, "Current Recommendations for Vaccines for Female Infertility Patients: A Committee Opinion," *Fertility and Sterility* 110, no. 5 (2018): 838–841.

21. American Society for Reproductive Medicine, "Current Recommendations for Vaccines for Female Infertility Patients."

22. J. M. Bieniek et al., "Influence of Increasing Body Mass Index on Semen and Reproductive Hormonal Parameters in a Multi-Institutional Cohort of Subfertile Men," *Fertility and Sterility* 106, no. 5 (2016): 1070–1075, https://doi.org/10.1016/j.fertnstert.2016.06.041.

23. L. Rato et al., "High-Energy Diets: A Threat for Male Fertility?" *Obesity Reviews* 15 (2014): 996–1007.

24. D. Vaamonde et al., "Physically Active Men Show Better Semen Parameters and Hormone Values than Sedentary Men," *European Journal of Applied Physiology* 112 (2012): 3267–3273.

25. J. T. Pajarinen and P. J. Karhunen, "Spermatogenic Arrest and 'Sertoli Cell-Only' Syndrome — Common Alcohol-Induced Disorders of the Human Testis," *International Journal of Andrology* 17, no. 6 (1994): 292–299.

26. K. R. Muthusami and P. Chinnaswamy, "Effect of Chronic Alcoholism on Male Fertility Hormones and Semen Quality," *Fertility and Sterility* 84, no. 4 (2005): 919–924.

27. M. L. Hansen et al., "Does Last Week's Alcohol Intake Affect Semen Quality or Reproductive Hormones? A Cross-Sectional Study Among Healthy Young Danish Men," *Reproductive Toxicology* 34, no. 3 (2012): 457–462.

28. M. Borgerding and H. Klus, "Analysis of Complex Mixtures — Cigarette Smoke," *Experimental and Toxicologic Pathology* 57, Suppl. 1 (2005): 43–73.

29. J. Jurasovic et al., "Semen Quality and Reproductive Endocrine Function with Regard to Blood Cadmium in Croatian Male Subjects," *Biometals* 17, no. 6 (2004): 735–743.

30. P. M. Zavos et al., "An Electron Microscope Study of the Axonemal Ultrastructure in Human Spermatozoa from Male Smokers and Nonsmokers," *Fertility and Sterility* 69, no. 3 (1998): 430.

31. V. Shrivastava et al., "Cigarette Smoke Affects Posttranslational Modifications and Inhibits Capacitation-Induced Changes in Human Sperm Proteins," *Reproductive Toxicology* 43 (2014): 125–129.

32. L. Peng et al., "Unraveling the Link: Environmental Tobacco Smoke Exposure and Its Impact on Infertility Among American Women (18–50 Years)," *Frontiers in Public Health* 12 (2024): 1358290, https://doi.org/10.3389/fpubh.2024.1358290.

33. S. S. du Plessis et al., "Marijuana, Phytocannabinoids, the Endocannabinoid System, and Male Fertility," *Journal of Assisted Reproduction and Genetics* 32, no. 11 (2015): 1575–1588.

34. R. C. Kolodny et al., "Depression of Plasma Testosterone Levels After Chronic Intensive Marihuana Use," *New England Journal of Medicine* 290, no. 16 (1974): 872–874.

35. A. A. Pacey et al., "Modifiable and Non-Modifiable Risk Factors for Poor Sperm Morphology," *Human Reproduction* 29, no. 8 (2014): 1629–1636.

CHAPTER 6 — SUPPLEMENTS THAT PROVIDE THE EXTRA VROOM

1. N. B. Duerbeck et al., "Prenatal Vitamins: What Is in the Bottle?" *Obstetrical and Gynecological Survey* 69, no. 12 (2014): 777–788.

2. M. Vidmar Golja et al., "Folate Insufficiency Due to MTHFR Deficiency Is Bypassed by 5-Methyltetrahydrofolate," *Journal of Clinical Medicine* 9, no. 9 (2020): 2836, DOI: 10.3390/jcm9092836.

3. R. Obeid et al., "Is 5-Methyltetrahydrofolate an Alternative to Folic Acid for the Prevention of Neural Tube Defects?" *Journal of Perinatal Medicine* 41, no. 5 (2013): 469–483, DOI: 10.1515/jpm-2012-0256.

4. Obeid et al., "Is 5-Methyltetrahydrofolate an Alternative to Folic Acid for the Prevention of Neural Tube Defects?"

5. Vidmar Golja et al., "Folate Insufficiency Due to MTHFR Deficiency Is Bypassed by 5-Methyltetrahydrofolate."

6. K. Neha et al., "Medicinal Prospects of Antioxidants: A Review," *European Journal of Medicinal Chemistry* 178 (2019): 687–704.

7. B. Brown and C. Wright, "Safety and Efficacy of Supplements in Pregnancy," *Nutrition Reviews* 78, no. 10 (2020): 813–826.

8. G. Morgante et al., "COS Physiopathology and Vitamin D Deficiency: Biological Insights and Perspectives for Treatment," *Journal of Clinical Medicine* 11, no. 15 (2022): 4509, DOI: 10.3390/jcm11154509.

9. Morgante et al., "COS Physiopathology and Vitamin D Deficiency."

10. C. Palacios et al., "Vitamin D Supplementation for Women During Pregnancy," *Cochrane Database of Systematic Reviews* 7, no. 7 (2019): CD008873, DOI: 10.1002/14651858.CD008873.pub4.

11. Brown and Wright, "Safety and Efficacy of Supplements in Pregnancy."

12. E. Larqué et al., "Omega 3 Fatty Acids, Gestation, and Pregnancy Outcomes," *British Journal of Nutrition* 107 Suppl. S2: S77–S84 (2012), DOI: 10.1017/S0007114512001481.

13. M. P. Judge et al., "Maternal Consumption of a Docosahexaenoic Acid-Containing Functional Food During Pregnancy: Benefit for Infant Performance on Problem-Solving But Not on Recognition Memory Tasks at Age 9 Mo.," *American Journal of Clinical Nutrition* 85 (2007): 1572–1577, DOI: 10.1093/ajcn/85.6.1572.

14. S. F. Olsen et al., "Fish Oil Intake Compared with Olive Oil Intake in Late Pregnancy and Asthma in the Offspring: 16 Years of Registry-Based Follow-up from a Randomized Controlled Trial," *American Journal of Clinical Nutrition* 88 (2008): 167–175, DOI: 10.1093/ajcn/88.1.167.

15. D. Swanson et al., "Omega-3 Fatty Acids EPA and DHA: Health Benefits Throughout Life," *Advances in Nutrition* 3, no. 1 (2008): 1–7, DOI: 10.3945/an.111.000893.

16. B. Koletzko et al. and World Association of Perinatal Medicine Dietary Guidelines Working Group, "The Roles of Long-Chain Polyunsaturated Fatty Acids in Pregnancy, Lactation, and Infancy: Review of Current

Knowledge and Consensus Recommendations," *Journal of Perinatal Medicine* 36, no. 1 (2008): 5–14, DOI: 10.1515/jpm.2008.001.

17. Y. Bentov et al., "The Contribution of Mitochondrial Function to Reproductive Aging," *Journal of Assisted Reproduction and Genetics* 28 (2011): 773–783.

18. D. R. Meldrum et al., "Aging and the Environment Affect Gamete and Embryo Potential: Can We Intervene?" *Fertility and Sterility* 195, no. 3 (2016): 548–559.

19. E. A. Schon et al., "Chromosomal Nondisjunction in Human Oocytes: Is There a Mitochondrial Connection?" *Human Reproduction* 15, Suppl. 2 (2000): 160–172.

20. Y. Bentov et al., "The Use of Mitochondrial Nutrients to Improve Outcome in Infertility in Older Patients," *Fertility and Sterility* 93 (2010): 272–275.

21. A. Ben-Meir et al., "Coenzyme Q10 Restores Oocyte Mitochondrial Function and Fertility During Reproductive Aging," *Aging Cell* 14 (2015): 887–895.

22. S. Hua et al., "Effects of Granulosa Cell Mitochondria Transfer on the Early Development of Bovine Embryos In Vitro," *Cloning and Stem Cells* 9, no. 2 (2007): 237–246.

23. Y. Bentov et al., "Coenzyme Q10 Supplementation and Oocyte Aneuploidy in Women Undergoing IVF-ICSI Treatment," *Clinical and Medical Insights: Reproductive Health* 8 (2014): 31–36.

24. L. Ma et al., "Coenzyme Q10 Supplementation of the Human Oocyte In Vitro Maturation Reduces Postmeiotic Aneuploidies," *Fertility and Sterility* 114, no. 2 (2020): 331–337.

25. Y. Xu et al., "Pretreatment with Coenzyme Q10 Improves Ovarian Response and Embryo Quality in Low-Prognosis Young Women with Decreased Ovarian Reserve: A Randomized Controlled Trial," *Reproductive Biology and Endocrinology* 16, no. 1 (2018): 29, DOI: 10.1186/s12958-018 -0343-0.

26. W. Yong et al., "Roles of Melatonin in the Field of Reproductive Medicine," *Biomedicine and Pharmacotherapy* 144 (2021): 112001, https://doi .org/10.1016/j.biopha.2021.112001.

27. R. J. Reiter et al., "Aging-Related Ovarian Failure and Infertility: Melatonin to the Rescue," *Antioxidants* 12, no. 3 (2023): 695, https://doi.org /10.3390/antiox12030695.

28. A. Brzezinski et al., "Melatonin in Human Preovulatory Follicular Fluid," *Journal of Clinical Endocrinology and Metabolism* 64, no. 4 (1987): 865–867, https://doi.org/10.1210/jcem-64-4-865; Y. Urata et al., "Melatonin Induces Gamma-Glutamylcysteine Synthetase Mediated by Activator Protein-1 in Human Vascular Endothelial Cells," *Free Radical Biology & Medicine* 27, nos. 7–8 (1999): 838–847, https://doi.org/10.1016/s0891-5849(99)00131-8.

29. H. Tamura et al., "Melatonin Regulates Female Reproduction," *Journal of Obstetrics and Gynaecology Research* 40 (2014): 1–11, https://doi.org/10.1111/jog.12177.

30. Yong et al., "Roles of Melatonin in the Field of Reproductive Medicine."

31. J. Tong et al., "Melatonin Levels in Follicular Fluid as Markers for IVF Outcomes and Predicting Ovarian Reserve," *Reproduction* 153, no. 4 (1999): 443–451, https://doi.org/10.1530/REP-16-0641.

32. B. N. Jahromi et al., "Effect of Melatonin on the Outcome of Assisted Reproductive Technique Cycles in Women with Diminished Ovarian Reserve: A Double-Blinded Randomized Clinical Trial," *Iranian Journal of Medical Sciences* 42, no. 1 (2017): 73–78.

33. K. L. Hu et al., "Melatonin Application in Assisted Reproductive Technology: A Systematic Review and Meta-Analysis of Randomized Trials," *Frontiers in Endocrinology* 11 (2020): 160, https://doi.org/10.3389/fendo.2020.00160.

34. P. Rizzo et al., "Effect of the Treatment with Myo-Inositol Plus Folic Acid Plus Melatonin in Comparison with a Treatment with Myo-Inositol Plus Folic Acid on Oocyte Quality and Pregnancy Outcome in IVF Cycles: A Prospective Clinical Trial," *European Review for Medical and Pharmacological Sciences* 14 (2010): 555–561.

35. R. Agarwal et al., "Evaluation of Dehydroepiandrosterone Supplementation on Diminished Ovarian Reserve: A Randomized, Double-Blinded, Placebo-Controlled Study," *Journal of Obstetrics and Gynecology of India* 67, no. 2 (2017): 137–142.

36. R. E. Wierman and K. Kiseljak-Vassiliades, "Should Dehydroepiandrosterone Be Given to Women?" *Journal of Clinical Endocrinology and Metabolism* 107 (2022): 1679–1685.

37. L. Lin et al., "Dehydroepiandrosterone as a Potential Agent to Slow Down Ovarian Aging," *Journal of Obstetrics and Gynaecology Research* 43, no. 12 (2017): 1855–1862.

38. C. Li et al., "Dehydroepiandrosterone Shifts Energy Metabolism to Increase Mitochondrial Biogenesis in Female Fertility with Advancing Age," *Nutrients* 13 (2021): 2449.

39. Agarwal et al., "Evaluation of Dehydroepiandrosterone Supplementation on Diminished Ovarian Reserve"; J. Hyman et al., "DHEA Supplementation May Improve IVF Outcome in Poor Responders: A Mechanism," *European Journal of Obstetrics and Gynecology and Reproductive Biology* 168 (2013): 49–53.

40. M. Elprince et al., "Ovarian Stimulation After Dehydroepiandrosterone Supplementation in Poor Ovarian Reserve: A Randomized Clinical Trial," *Archives of Gynecology and Obstetrics* 302 (2020): 529–534; C. Chern et al., "Dehydroepiandrosterone (DHEA) Supplementation Improves In Vitro Fertilization Outcomes of Poor Ovarian Responders, Especially in Women with Low Serum Concentration of DHEA-S: A Retrospective Cohort Study," *Reproductive Biology and Endocrinology* 16 (2018): 90; Q. Hu et al., "The Effect of Dehydroepiandrosterone Supplementation on Ovarian Response Is Associated with Androgen Receptor in Diminished Ovarian Reserve Women," *Journal of Ovarian Research* 10 (2017): 32; J. Li et al., "A Meta-Analysis of Dehydroepiandrosterone Supplementation Among Women with Diminished Ovarian Reserve Undergoing In Vitro Fertilization or Intracytoplasmic Sperm Injection," *International Journal of Gynecology and Obstetrics* 131 (2015): 240–245.

41. Li et al., "A Meta-Analysis of Dehydroepiandrosterone Supplementation Among Women with Diminished Ovarian Reserve Undergoing In Vitro Fertilization or Intracytoplasmic Sperm Injection."

42. F. Caprio et al., "Myo-Inositol Therapy for Poor-Responders During IVF: A Prospective Controlled Observational Trial," *Journal of Ovarian Research* 8 (2015): 37.

43. A. S. Lagana et al., "Myo-Inositol Supplementation Reduces the Amount of Gonadotropins and Length of Ovarian Stimulation in Women Undergoing IVF: A Systematic Review and Meta-Analysis of Randomized Controlled Trials," *Archives of Gynecology and Obstetrics* 298 (2018): 675–684; A. Agrawal et al., "Comparison of Metformin Plus Myoinositol vs Metformin Alone in PCOS Women Undergoing Ovulation Induction Cycles: Randomized Controlled Trial," *Gynecological Endocrinology* 35 (2019): 511–514; B. Lesoine and P. A. Regidor, "Prospective Randomized Study on the Influence of Myoinositol in PCOS Women Undergoing IVF in the Improvement of Oocyte Quality, Fertilization Rate, and Embryo Quality," *International*

Journal of Endocrinology, 2016, 4378507, https://doi.org/10.1155/2016 /4378507.

44. M. Bizzarri et al., "Myo-Inositol and D-Chiro-Inositol as Modulators of Ovary Steroidogenesis: A Narrative Review," *Nutrients* 15, no. 8 (2023): 1875.

45. P. G. Artini et al., "Endocrine and Clinical Effects of Myo-Inositol Administration in Polycystic Ovary Syndrome: A Randomized Study," *Gynecological Endocrinology* 29 (2013): 375–379.

46. P. Prabhakar et al., "Impact of Myoinositol with Metformin and Myoinositol Alone in Infertile PCOS Women Undergoing Ovulation Induction Cycles — Randomized Controlled Trial," *Gynecological Endocrinology* 37, no. 4 (2021): 332–336, https://doi.org/10.1080/09513590.2020.1810657; Agrawal et al., "Comparison of Metformin Plus Myoinositol vs Metformin Alone in PCOS Women Undergoing Ovulation Induction Cycles."

47. Prabhakar et al., "Impact of Myoinositol with Metformin and Myo-inositol Alone in Infertile PCOS Women Undergoing Ovulation Induction Cycles"; Agrawal et al., "Comparison of Metformin Plus Myoinositol vs Metformin Alone in PCOS Women Undergoing Ovulation Induction Cycles"; K. Rajasekaran et al., "Myoinositol Versus Metformin Pretreatment in GnRH-Antagonist Cycle for Women with PCOS Undergoing IVF: A Double-Blinded Randomized Controlled Study," *Gynecological Endocrinology* 38, no. 2 (2022): 140–147; F. Seyedoshohadaei et al., "Myoinositol Effect on Pregnancy Outcomes in Infertile Women Undergoing In Vitro Fertilization/Intracytoplasmic Sperm Injection: A Double Blind RCT," *International Journal of Reproductive BioMedicine* 20 (2022): 643–650.

48. C. A. Hogarth and M. D. Griswold, "The Key Role of Vitamin A in Spermatogenesis," *Journal of Clinical Investigation* 120, no. 4 (2010): 956–962, https://doi.org/10.1172/JCI41303.

49. S. Ahmadi et al., "Antioxidant Supplements and Semen Parameters: An Evidence Based Review," *International Journal of Reproductive Biomedicine* 14, no. 12 (2016): 729–736.

50. E. Y. Ko and E. S. Sabanegh, "The Role of Nutraceuticals in Male Fertility," *Urology Clinics of North America* 41, no. 1 (2014): 181–193, DOI: 10.1016/j.ucl.2013.08.003.

51. Ahmadi et al., "Antioxidant Supplements and Semen Parameters: An Evidence Based Review."

52. M. Kuchakulla et al., "A Systematic Review and Evidence-Based Analysis of Ingredients in Popular Male Fertility Supplements," *Urology* 136 (2020): 133–141, DOI: 10.1016/j.urology.2019.11.007.

53. R. Jannatifar et al., "Effects of N-Acetyl-Cysteine Supplementation on Sperm Quality, Chromatin Integrity and Level of Oxidative Stress in Infertile Men," *Reproductive Biology and Endocrinology* 17, no. 1 (2019): 24, https://doi.org/10.1186/s12958-019-0468-9.

54. Y. Lv et al., "Melatonin Protects Mouse Spermatogonial Stem Cells Against Hexavalent Chromium-Induced Apoptosis and Epigenetic Histone Modification," *Toxicology and Applied Pharmacology* 340 (2018): 30–38, https://doi.org/10.1016/j.taap.2017.12.017.

CHAPTER 9 — EMBRYO TRANSFERS: FRESH START OR ICE-COLD SURPRISE

1. B. S. Shapiro et al., "Matched-Cohort Comparison of Single-Embryo Transfers in Fresh and Frozen-Thawed Embryo Transfer Cycles," *Fertility and Sterility* 99 (2013): 389–392; J. Z. Chen et al., "Fresh vs Frozen Embryos for Infertility in the Polycystic Ovarian Syndrome," *New England Journal of Medicine* 375 (2016): 523–533; K. Devine et al., "Intramuscular Progesterone Optimizes Live Birth from a Programmed Frozen Embryo Transfer: A Randomized Clinical Trial," *Fertility and Sterility* 116 (2021): 633–643.

2. P. Bortoletto et al., "Association Between Programmed Frozen Embryo Transfer and Hypertensive Disorders of Pregnancy," *Fertility and Sterility* 118 (2022): 839–848.

3. Y. C. Hsieh et al., "Association Between Estradiol Levels in Early Pregnancy and Risk of Preeclampsia After Frozen Embryo Transfer," *Frontiers in Endocrinology* 14 (2023): 1223181.

4. U. B. Wennerholm et al., "Perinatal Outcomes of Children Born After Frozen-Thawed Embryo Transfer: A Nordic Cohort Study from the CoNARTaS group," *Human Reproduction* 28 (2013): 2545–2553.

CHAPTER 10 — IVF: IT'S A NUMBERS GAME

1. H. Levine et al., "Temporal Trends in Sperm Count: A Systemic Review and Meta-Regression Analysis," *Human Reproduction Update* 23, no. 6 (2017): 1–14.

2. N. Punjani et al., "The Use of Fresh Compared to Frozen Ejaculated Sperm Has No Impact on Fresh Embryo Transfer Cycle Reproductive Outcomes," *Journal of Assisted Reproduction and Genetics* 39 (2022): 1409–1414.

3. P. N. Schlegel, "We Are Giving the Wrong Patient Instructions for Semen Analysis Before Assisted Reproductive Technology," *Fertility and Sterility* 23 (2023): 426–427.

4. J. Kalsi et al., "Analysis of the Outcome of Intracytoplasmic Sperm Injection Using Fresh or Frozen Sperm," *British Journal of Urology International* 107 (2010): 1124–1128.

5. T. Peng et al., "Gonadotropins Treatment Prior to Microdissection Testicular Sperm Extraction in Non-Obstructive Azoospermia: A Single-Center Cohort Study," *Reproductive Biology and Endocrinology* 20 (2022): 61.

6. G. Grande et al., "FSH Therapy in Male Factor Infertility: Evidence and Factors Which Might Predict the Response," *Life* 14 (2024): 969; J. Fink et al., "Human Chorionic Gonadotropin Treatment: A Viable Option for Management of Secondary Hypogonadism and Male Infertility," *Expert Review of Endocrinology and Metabolism* 16 (2021): 1–8.

7. B. Guo et al., "Efficacy and Safety of Letrozole or Anastrozole in the Treatment of Male Infertility with Low Testosterone-Estradiol Ratio: A Meta-Analysis and Systematic Review," *Andrology* 10 (2022): 894–909.

8. M. Huijben et al., "Clomiphene Citrate for Male Infertility: A Systematic Review and Meta-Analysis," *Andrology* 11 (2022): 987–996.

9. A. D. Coviello et al., "Intratesticular Testosterone Concentrations Comparable with Serum Levels Are Not Sufficient to Maintain Normal Sperm Production in Men Receiving a Hormonal Contraceptive Regimen," *Journal of Andrology* 25 (2004): 931–938.

10. O. O. Oduwole et al., "Constitutively Active Follicle-Stimulating Hormone Receptor Enables Androgen-Independent Spermatogenesis," *Journal of Clinical Investigation* 128, no. 5 (2018): 1787–1792.

11. A. Hussein et al., "Optimization of Spermatogenesis-Regulating Hormones in Patients with Non-Obstructive Azoospermia and Its Impact on Sperm Retrieval: A Multicenter Study," *British Journal of Urology International* 111 (2013): E110–114.

12. Hussein et al., "Optimization of Spermatogenesis-Regulating Hormones in Patients with Non-Obstructive Azoospermia and Its Impact on Sperm Retrieval."

CHAPTER 13 — IT'S COLD IN HERE: GETTING READY FOR FROZEN EMBRYO TRANSFER

1. Z. O. Amarin and B. R. Obeidat, "Bed Rest Versus Free Mobilisation Following Embryo Transfer: A Prospective Randomised Study," *British Journal of Obstetrics and Gynecology* 111, no. 11 (2004): 1273–1276.

2. M. J. Lambers et al., "Ultrasonographic Evidence That Bedrest After Embryo Transfer Is Useless," *Gynecologic and Obstetric Investigation* 68, no. 2 (2009): 122–126.

CHAPTER 15 — EGG-CELLENT INSURANCE: THE SCIENCE OF FREEZING YOUR FUTURE

1. Ethics Committee of the American Society for Reproductive Medicine, "Planned Oocyte Cryopreservation to Preserve Future Reproductive Potential: An Ethics Committee Opinion," *Fertility and Sterility* 121 (2024): 604–612.

2. Practice Committee of the American Society for Reproductive Medicine, "Evidence-Based Outcomes After Oocyte Cryopreservation for Donor Oocyte In Vitro Fertilization and Planned Oocyte Cryopreservation: A Guideline," *Fertility and Sterility* 116 (2021): 36–47.

3. T. B. Mesen et al., "Optimal Timing for Elective Egg Freezing," *Fertility and Sterility* 103 (2015): 1551–1556.

4. C. Meernik et al., "Fertility Preservation and Financial Hardship Among Adolescent and Young Adult Women with Cancer," *Cancer Epidemiology Biomarkers Prevention* 31 (2022): 1043–1051.

5. S. J. Chua et al., "Age-Related Natural Fertility Outcomes in Women Over 35 Years: A Systematic Review and Individual Participant Meta-Analysis," *Human Reproduction* 35 (2020): 1808–1820.

6. Ethics Committee of the American Society for Reproductive Medicine, "Planned Oocyte Cryopreservation to Preserve Future Reproductive Potential."

7. Practice Committee of the American Society for Reproductive Medicine, "Evidence-Based Outcomes After Oocyte Cryopreservation for Donor Oocyte In Vitro Fertilization and Planned Oocyte Cryopreservation."

8. Y. T. Su et al., "Age Is a Major Prognosticator in Extremely Low Oocyte Retrieval Cycles," *Taiwanese Journal of Obstetrics and Gynecology* 56 (2017): 175–180.

9. M. Tatickova et al., "The Ultrastructural Nature of Human Oocytes' Cytoplasm Abnormalities and the Role of Cytoskeleton Dysfunction," *F&S Science* 4, no. 4 (2023): 267–278.

10. R. J. Rodgers et al., "The Safety and Efficacy of Controlled Ovarian Hyperstimulation for Fertility Preservation in Women with Early Breast Cancer: A Systematic Review," *Human Reproduction* 32 (2017): 1033–1045.

11. Rodgers et al., "The Safety and Efficacy of Controlled Ovarian Hyperstimulation for Fertility Preservation in Women with Early Breast Cancer."

12. Practice Committee of the American Society for Reproductive Medicine, "Fertility Preservation in Patients Undergoing Gonadotoxic Therapy or Gonadectomy: A Committee Opinion," *Fertility and Sterility* 112, no. 6 (2019): 1022–1033.

13. Rodgers et al., "The Safety and Efficacy of Controlled Ovarian Hyperstimulation for Fertility Preservation in Women with Early Breast Cancer."

14. Practice Committee of the American Society for Reproductive Medicine, "Fertility Preservation in Patients Undergoing Gonadotoxic Therapy or Gonadectomy"; J. J. Chan and E. T. Wang, "Oncofertility for Women with Gynecologic Malignancies," *Gynecologic Oncology* 144 (2017): 631–635.

15. Chan and Wang, "Oncofertility for Women with Gynecologic Malignancies."

16. Practice Committee of the American Society for Reproductive Medicine, "Fertility Preservation in Patients Undergoing Gonadotoxic Therapy or Gonadectomy."

17. E. Fraison et al., "Live Birth Rate After Female Fertility Preservation for Cancer or Haematopoietic Stem Cell Transplantation: A Systematic Review and Meta-Analysis of the Three Main Techniques; Embryo, Oocyte and Ovarian Tissue Cryopreservation," *Human Reproduction* 38 (2023): 489–502.

18. A. Volodarsky-Perel et al., "Effects of Cancer Stage and Grade on Fertility Preservation Outcome and Ovarian Stimulation Response," *Human Reproduction* 34 (2019): 530–538; M. M. Dolmans and J. Donnez, "Fertility Preservation in Women for Medical and Social Reasons: Oocytes vs Ovarian Tissue," *Best Practice & Research Clinical Obstetrics and Gynaecology* 70 (2021): 63–80.

19. Chan and Wang, "Oncofertility for Women with Gynecologic Malignancies"; Volodarsky-Perel et al., "Effects of Cancer Stage and Grade on Fertility Preservation Outcome and Ovarian Stimulation Response"; Dolmans and Donnez, "Fertility Preservation in Women for Medical and Social Reasons."

20. Meernik et al., "Fertility Preservation and Financial Hardship Among Adolescent and Young Adult Women with Cancer."

21. Practice Committee of the American Society for Reproductive Medicine, "Fertility Preservation in Patients Undergoing Gonadotoxic Therapy or Gonadectomy."

22. Dolmans and Donnez, "Fertility Preservation in Women for Medical and Social Reasons."

23. R. B. Gilchrist and J. Smitz, "Oocyte In Vitro Maturation: Physiologic Basis and Application to Clinical Practice," *Fertility and Sterility* 119 (2023): 524–539; Practice Committee of the American Society for Reproductive Medicine, Practice Committee of the Society of Biologists and Technologists, and Practice Committee of the Society for Assisted Reproductive Technology, "In Vitro Maturation: A Committee Opinion," *Fertility and Sterility* 115 (2021): 298–304.

24. J. Cadenas et al., "Future Potential of In Vitro Maturation Including Fertility Preservation," *Fertility and Sterility* 119 (2023): 550–559.

25. Fraison et al., "Live Birth Rate After Female Fertility Preservation for Cancer or Haematopoietic Stem Cell Transplantation"; H. Khattak et al., "Fresh and Cryopreserved Ovarian Tissue Transplantation for Preserving Reproductive and Endocrine Function: A Systematic Review and Individual Patient Meta-Analysis," *Human Reproduction Update* 28 (2022): 400–416.

26. Practice Committee of the American Society for Reproductive Medicine, "Fertility Preservation in Patients Undergoing Gonadotoxic Therapy or Gonadectomy."

27. M. L. Metzger et al., "Female Reproductive Health After Childhood, Adolescent and Young Adult Cancers: Guidelines for the Assessment and Management of Female Reproductive Complications," *Journal of Clinical Oncology* 31 (2013): 1239–1247.

CHAPTER 16 — LEAN ON ME: EGG, SPERM, AND EMBRYO DONORS

1. S. Matsuzaki et al., "Obstetric Characteristics and Outcomes of Gestational Carrier Pregnancies: A Systematic Review and Meta-Analysis," *Obstetrics and Gynecology* 7 (2024): e2422634; R. M. Mortimer et al., "Predictors of Gamete Donation: A Cross Sectional Survey Study," *Assisted Reproduction Technologies* 41 (2024): 2327–2336; Practice Committee of the American Society for Reproductive Medicine, "Repetitive Oocyte Donation: A Committee Opinion," *Fertility and Sterility* 113 (2020): 1150–1153.

2. Practice Committee of the American Society for Reproductive Medicine and the Practice Committee for the Society for Assisted Reproductive Technology, "Guidance Regarding Gamete and Embryo Donation," *Fertility and Sterility* 115 (2021): 1395–1410.

3. Ethics Committee of the American Society for Reproductive Medicine, "Ethical Issues in Oocyte Banking for Nonautologous Use: An Ethics Committee Opinion," *Fertility and Sterility* 116 (2021): 644–650.

4. Practice Committee of the American Society for Reproductive Medicine and the Practice Committee for the Society for Assisted Reproductive Technology, "Guidance Regarding Gamete and Embryo Donation."

5. Ethics and Practice Committees of the American Society for Reproductive Medicine, "Updated Terminology for Gamete and Embryo Donors: Directed (Identified) to Replace 'Known' and Non Identified to Replace 'Anonymous': A Committee Opinion," *Fertility and Sterility* 118 (2022): 75–78.

6. C. De Jonge and C. L. R. Barratt, "Gamete Donation: A Question of Anonymity," *Fertility and Sterility* 85 (2006): 500–501.

7. D. H. Siegel, "Open Adoption: Adoptive Parents' Reactions Two Decades Later," *Social Work* 58 (2013): 43–52; R. Burke et al., "How Do Individuals Who Were Conceived Through the Use of Donor Technologies Feel About the Nature of Their Conception?," Harvard Medical School Center for Bioethics, April 1, 2021, https://bioethics.hms.harvard.edu/journal/donor-technology; O. B. A. Van den Akker et al., "Expectations and Experiences of Gamete Donors and Donor-Conceived Adults Searching for Genetic Relatives Using DNA Linking Through a Voluntary Register," *Human Reproduction* 30 (2015): 111–121.

8. R. H. Farr et al., "Adoptees' Contact with Birth Parents in Emergent Adulthood: The Role of Adoption Communication and Attachment to Adoptive Parents," *Family Process* 53 (2014): 656–671.

9. E. Thorup et al., "Same-Sex Mothers' Experience of Equal Treatment, Parenting Stress, and Disclosure to Offspring: A Population Based Study of Parenthood Following Identity-Release Sperm Donation," *Human Reproduction* 37 (2022): 2589–2598.

10. Van den Akker et al., "Expectations and Experiences of Gamete Donors and Donor-Conceived Adults Searching for Genetic Relatives Using DNA Linking Through a Voluntary Register."

11. M. Tatickova et al., "The Ultrastructural Nature of Human Oocytes' Cytoplasm Abnormalities and the Role of Cytoskeleton Dysfunction," *F&S Science* 4, no. 4 (2023): 267–278.

12. M. L. Eisenberg et al., "Male Infertility Primer," *Nature Reviews Disease Primers* 9 (2023): 49–61.

13. J. C. Lee et al., "Embryo Donation: National Trends and Outcomes, 2004–2019," *American Journal of Obstetrics and Gynecology* 228 (2023): 318. e1–318.e7.

CHAPTER 17 — AN OVEN FOR THE BUN: GESTATIONAL CARRIERS

1. Practice Committee of the American Society for Reproductive Medicine, "Recommendations for Practices Using Gestational Carriers: A Committee Opinion," *Fertility and Sterility* 118 (2022): 65–74.

2. Ethics Committee of the American Society for Reproductive Medicine, "Consideration of the Gestational Carrier: An Ethics Committee Opinion," *Fertility and Sterility* 119 (2023): 583–588.

3. Ethics Committee of the American Society for Reproductive Medicine, "Consideration of the Gestational Carrier."

4. Practice Committee of the American Society for Reproductive Medicine, "Recommendations for Practices Using Gestational Carriers."

CHAPTER 18 — LGBTQIA+ FAMILY-BUILDING

1. PFLAG, "PFLAG National Glossary," accessed January 18, 2025, https://pflag.org/glossary.

2. E. V. Lemos et al., "Healthcare Expenses Associated with Multiple vs Singleton Pregnancies in the United States," *American Journal of Obstetrics and Gynecology* 209 (2013): 586:e1–e11.

3. American College of Obstetricians and Gynecologists, "Multifetal Pregnancy Reduction: Committee Opinion No. 719," *Obstetrics and Gynecology* 130 (2017): e158–e163.

4. A. R. Schwartz and M. B. Moravek, "Reproductive Potential and Fertility Preservation in Transgender and Nonbinary Individuals," *Current Opinion in Obstetrics and Gynecology* 33 (2021): 327–334.

5. Schwartz and Moravek, "Reproductive Potential and Fertility Preservation in Transgender and Nonbinary Individuals"; M. B. Moravek et al., "Impact of Exogenous Testosterone on Reproduction in Transgender Men," *Endocrinology* 161 (2020): 1–13; S. C. Cromack et al., "Oocyte Cryopreservation in Transgender and Gender-Diverse Individuals with or Without Prior Testosterone Use," *Obstetrics and Gynecology* 144 (2024): e121–e124.

6. M. B. Moravek et al., "Impact of Exogenous Testosterone on Reproduction in Transgender Men," *Endocrinology* 161 (2020): 1–13.

7. H. M. Kinnear and M. B. Moravek, "Reproductive Capacity After Gender Affirming Testosterone Therapy," *Human Reproduction* 38 (2023): 1872–1880.

CHAPTER 19 — BEYOND INFERTILITY: THE OTHER REASONS FOR CHOOSING IVF

1. H. B. Ford and D. J. Schust, "Recurrent Pregnancy Loss: Etiology, Diagnosis, and Therapy," *Reviews in Obstetrics and Gynecology* 2 (2009): 76–83; C. R. Jaslow et al., "Diagnostic Factors Identified in 1020 Women with Two Versus Three or More Recurrent Pregnancy Losses," *Fertility and Sterility* 93, no. 4 (2010): 1234–1243, https://doi.org/10.1016/j.fertnstert.2009.01.166; M. D. Stephenson, "Frequency of Factors Associated with Habitual Abortion in 197 Couples," *Fertility and Sterility* 66, no. 1 (1996): 24–29, https://doi .org/10.1016/j.fertnstert.2009.01.166.

2. M. D. Stephenson et al., "Cytogenetic Analysis of Miscarriages from Couples with Recurrent Miscarriage: A Case-Control Study," *Human Repro-duction* 17, no. 2 (2002): 446–451, https://doi.org/10.1093/humrep/17.2.446; Jaslow et al., "Diagnostic Factors Identified in 1020 Women with Two Versus Three or More Recurrent Pregnancy Losses."

3. Jaslow et al., "Diagnostic Factors Identified in 1020 Women with Two Versus Three or More Recurrent Pregnancy Losses"; M. D. Stephenson, "Fre-quency of Factors Associated with Habitual Abortion in 197 Couples," *Fertil-ity and Sterility* 66, no. 1 (1996): 24–29.

4. S. J. Bhatt et al., "Pregnancy Outcomes Following In Vitro Fertiliza-tion Frozen Embryo Transfer (IVF-FET) with or Without Preimplantation Genetic Testing for Aneuploidy (PGT-A) in Women with Recurrent Preg-nancy Loss (RPL): A SART-CORS Study," *Human Reproduction* 36, no. 8 (2021): 2339–2344.

INDEX

· · · · · · · · · · · · · · · · ·

Note: Italic page numbers refer to illustrations.

Index

Index

Index

IVF medications *(cont.)*
  information on, 37
  injection instructions and, 17, 40, 44
  injection process and, 5, 6, 13, 17, 44, 51, 55
  ovulation preventers, 43, 51–52
  ovulation suppressors, 47, 48, 51–53
  preparation meds, 43, 46, 47–48
  protocols for, 117–123
  side effects of, 43, 55–57
  specialty pharmacies for, 115–117
  stimulation medications, 43, 45, 46–47, 48, 49–53, 115–117
  trigger medications, 43, 47, 53–54, 122–123
IVF monitoring visits, 37
IVF nurses, 40, 44
IVF process, 1–8, 16–18, 41, 56–57
IVF stimulation
  egg retrieval and, 35, 122, 123
  endometrial preparation and, 140
  estradiol levels and, 119–120
  estrogen priming cycle and, 118–119
  medication protocols, 117–123
  medications for, 43, 45, 46–47, 48, 49–53, 115–117
  oncofertility and, 225–227
  progesterone production and, 55–56, 123, 139–140, 141
  tolerance levels for, 128
  trigger shot and, 122–123, 139, 140
  vaginal ultrasounds and, 119, 120–121
IVF success estimator, 37

karotypes, 238
karyotype analysis, 178

labor complications, 90–91
legal issues. *See* reproductive law
letrozole, 47, 51, 186, 195, 226–227
leuprolide
  for cancer patients, 229
  day 21 leuprolide, 46, 47, 48, 50, 52, 53, 117, 119
  for frozen embryo transfers, 189, 260
  leuprolide trigger, 46, 47, 53, 72, 117, 122, 123, 142, 186
  long leuprolide protocol, 54

microdose leuprolide flare, 46–47, 48, 50, 117–118, 119
levothyroxine, 75
Leydig cells, 96
LGBTQIA+ population
  clinic choice and, 264–265
  donor-GC cycles in AMAB couples, 269–272
  family-building and, 263, 269, 276
  financial costs and, 269–270
  name verifications for, 265
  reciprocal IVF in AFAB couples, 35–36, 264, 265–269
  sperm and egg donation and, 232
  terms related to, 264, 265
  trans patients, 274–276
LH (luteinizing hormone)
  levels of, 21, 45, 55, 110, 123
  men's level of, 154, 155, 156
  production of, 45, 46, 48, 49, 69
  release of, 47, 50, 69, 186
  suppression of release, 119
LH surge, 45, 52, 53, 54, 72, 139, 146
lifestyle choices, 81–85, 91–96, 187–188
low birth weight, 64–65, 71, 74, 83, 86, 102, 147–148
lupus, 29, 66

male couples, 35, 249, 269–272
marijuana, 81, 82, 84–85, 96, 188
maternal deaths, 60, 91
maternal weight, 85–88, 90–91, 101
meiosis, 28, 105, 151, 152, 159, *170*, 171–172
melanoma, 283
melatonin, 105–107, 110–111
men, 68, 87, 94–96
menotropins, 46, 49–50, 69
menstrual cycle, 48, 136, 169, 183, 194
mental health, 20, 32–33, 59, 69–72, 200, 209, 212
metformin, 78–79, 87, 95
microprolactinoma, 77
miscarriages. *See also* recurrent pregnancy loss
  age and, 28, 172
  alprazolam and, 71
  autoimmune diseases and, 66, 74

Index

ABOUT THE AUTHORS

Abby Eblen, MD, MSHS, is board certified in obstetrics and gynecology and in reproductive endocrinology and infertility. In 2022 and 2023, she was named as one of Nashville's Top Docs by *Nashville Lifestyles* magazine. Her practice, Nashville Fertility Center, was named as the thirteenth-best fertility practice in the United States in 2023 by *Newsweek* magazine. She is currently an assistant professor for the University of Tennessee Nashville OB/GYN residency program.

Carrie Bedient, MD, is board certified in obstetrics and gynecology and in reproductive endocrinology and infertility. Dr. Bedient is the director of reproductive endocrinology and infertility at Mountain View OB/GYN residency and a clinical associate professor for the Kirk Kerkorian College of Medicine at the University of Nevada Las Vegas. She currently is a partner and director of egg donation at the Fertility Center of Las Vegas.

Susan Hudson, MD, MBA, is board certified in reproductive endocrinology and infertility and in obstetrics and gynecology. Dr. Hudson practices at Texas Fertility Center in New Braunfels and Corpus Christi, Texas. She currently serves as medical director for an Ovation-network andrology lab within her clinic. She served as chair for the Texas Medical Association Council on Practice Management Services from 2019 to 2021 and is an active member of the American Society for Reproductive Medicine and the Comal County Medical Society.

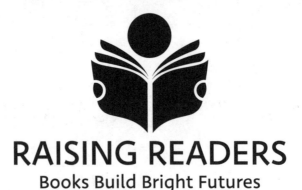

RAISING READERS
Books Build Bright Futures

Thank you for reading this book and for being a reader of books in general. As author, I am so grateful to share being part of a community of readers with y and I hope you will join me in passing our love of books on to the next generat of readers.

Did you know that reading for enjoyment is the single biggest predictor o child's future happiness and success?

More than family circumstances, parents' educational background, or incor reading impacts a child's future academic performance, emotional well-bei communication skills, economic security, ambition, and happiness.

Studies show that kids reading for enjoyment in the US is in rapid decline:

- In 2012, 53% of 9-year-olds read almost every day. Just 10 years later, in 2022, the number had fallen to 39%.
- In 2012, 27% of 13-year-olds read for fun daily. By 2023, that number was just 14%.

Together, we can commit to **Raising Readers** and change this trend. How?

- Read to children in your life daily.
- Model reading as a fun activity.
- Reduce screen time.
- Start a family, school, or community book club.
- Visit bookstores and libraries regularly.
- Listen to audiobooks.
- Read the book before you see the movie.
- Encourage your child to read aloud to a pet or stuffed animal.
- Give books as gifts.
- Donate books to families and communities in need.

Books build bright futures, and **Raising Readers** is our shared responsibility